American College of Surgeons
Deutsche Gesellschaft für Chirurgie

Joint Meeting

Munich 1968

Edited by

H. Bürkle de la Camp, F. Linder and M. Trede
Assisted by G. Kolig and K. Junghanns
Section on Gynecology edited by J. Zander

Special Reprint
of the
Gynecological Section

With 51 Figures

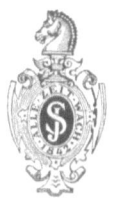

Springer-Verlag Berlin Heidelberg GmbH 1969

Proceedings of the Sectional Meeting of the American College of Surgeons in Cooperation with the Deutsche Gesellschaft für Chirurgie June 26—29, 1968, in Munich

These papers are reprinted from the full report of the Joint Meeting of the American College of Surgeons and the Deutsche Gesellschaft für Chirurgie, Munich, June 26—29, 1968, and published by Springer-Verlag Berlin · Heidelberg · New York 1969

ISBN 978-3-540-04402-4   ISBN 978-3-662-00828-7 (eBook)

DOI 10.1007/978-3-662-00828-7

Contents

Introduction, authors and titles of the other papers presented at this Meeting are listed below.

Introduction

This volume contains some hundred papers read before a Sectional Meeting of the American College of Surgeons held in conjunction with the German Surgical Society in Munich from 25th through 29th June 1968. The committee responsible for the scientific program, headed by WILLIAM P. LONGMIRE (Los Angeles) and FRITZ LINDER (Heidelberg) was able to obtain the cooperation of American and European experts in providing a survey of topical problems concerning general and special operative medicine. Thus the subjects range from general surgery with all its specialities, to traumatology and orthopedics, urology as well as gynecology. The response from our colleagues was most gratifying: More than 1200 surgeons from 33 nations, two-thirds of them from the United States and Canada, participated in this international exchange of information, which was supplemented by a series of panel discussions.

We wish to thank Springer-Verlag, Berlin-Heidelberg-New York for publishing these proceedings and thereby contributing to a world wide interest in the improvement of operative therapy. In addition our gratitude has to be expressed to many members of the Surgical Department of Heidelberg University who have given great support and enthusiasm to the preparation of this volume.

The Editors.

Contents

Physiology and Surgery of Peptic Ulcer

The Pancreas

Portal Hypertension

Surgery of Infants and Children

Plastic and Reconstructive Surgery

Operative Treatment of Fractures

Urologic Injuries

Renal Stones

Gynecology

X

List of Participants

ALKEN, C. E., Professor Dr. med., Director of the Urological University Hospital and Medical School of the University at Homburg/Saar

ALLGÖWER, M., M. D., F. A. C. S., Professor and Chairman of the Department of Surgery, University of Basel, Switzerland

AUSTEN, W. G., M. D., F. A. C. S., Professor of Surgery, Harvard Medical School, Boston

BAILEY, R. W., M. D., F. A. C. S., Professor of Surgery, Section of Orthopaedic Surgery, University of Michigan School of Medicine, Ann Arbor

BAUER, K. H., Professor Emeritus of Surgery, Delegate of the Board of Trustees, German Cancer Research Institute, Heidelberg

BEACHAM, W. D., M. D., F. A. C. S., Professor of Clinical Obstetrics and Gynecology, Tulane University School of Medicine, New Orleans

BISCHOFF, P., Dr., Professor of Urology and Chief, Department of Urology, St. Elizabeth Hospital and Children's Hospital of Hochallee, Hamburg

BLOCKER, T. G., JR., M. D., F. A. C. S., Professor of Surgery and Dean, University of Texas Medical Branch, Galveston

BORST, H.-G., M. D., Professor of Surgery and Director, Surgical University Hospital, Hannover

BOYES, J. H., M. D., F. A. C. S., Clinical Professor of Surgery, University of Southern California School of Medicine, Los Angeles

BRAMANN, C. VON, Dr. med., Specialist in Surgery, Berlin

BREWER, J. I., M. D., F. A. C. S., Professor of Obstetrics and Gynecology, Northwestern University Medical School, Chicago

BRICKER, E. M., M. D., F. A. C. S., Professor of Clinical Surgery, Washington University School of Medicine, St. Louis

BROSIG, W. J., Dr., Professor of Urology and Director, Urological University Clinic, Free University School of Medicine, Berlin

BUCK-GRAMCKO, D., Dr. med., Chief, Department of Hand Surgery, Traumatology Hospital, Hamburg-Bergedorf

BÜRKLE DE LA CAMP, H., Dr. med., Professor of Surgery and Secretary of the German Surgical Society, Dottingen

CAVE, E. F., M. D., F. A. C. S., Consulting Visiting Orthopaedic Surgeon, Massachusetts General Hospital, Boston

COCKETT, A. T. K., M. D., F. A. C. S., Associate Professor of Surgery/Urology, Harbor General Hospital, Torrance, California

COPE, O., M. D., F. A. C. S., Professor of Surgery, Harvard Medical School and Visiting Surgeon, Massachusetts General Hospital, Boston

CULP, D. A., M. D., F. A. C. S., Professor of Urology, State University of Iowa College of Medicine, Iowa City

D'AUBIGNE, R. MERLE, Prof. M. D., F. A. C. S. (Hon.), Professor of Orthopaedic Surgery, University of Paris

DETERLING, R. A., JR., M. D., F. A. C. S., Professor and Chairman, Department of Surgery, Tufts University School of Medicine, Boston

DINGMAN, R. O., M. D., F. A. C. S., Professor of Surgery and Head, Section of Plastic Surgery, University of Michigan School of Medicine, Ann Arbor

EKMAN, C.-A., M. D., Associate Professor, Surgical Department, University of Lund, Sweden

ERICSSON, N. O., M. D., Professor of Pediatric Urology, Karolinska Institute, Stockholm

FIKENTSCHER, R., Dr., Professor of Obstetrics and Gynecology and Director of the Hospital for Women No. 2 of the University of Munich

FREY, E. K., Professor Emeritus of Surgery, Munich

FUCHSIG, P., Dr., Professor of Surgery and Head of the First Surgical University Hospital, Vienna

GEORG, H., Dr., Lecturer in Surgery, University of Heidelberg School of Medicine and Chief, Department of Surgery, Municipal Hospital, Pforzheim

GEORGIADE, N. G., M. D., F. A. C. S., Professor of Plastic and Maxillofacial Surgery. Department of Surgery, Duke University School of Medicine, Durham

GERBODE, F. L. A., M. D., F. A. C. S., Clinical Professor of Surgery, Stanford University and University of California School of Medicine, San Francisco

GLENN, F., M. D., F. A. C. S., Professor of Surgery, Cornell University Medical College, New York

GÖGLER, E., Dr. med., Lecturer, Surgical University Hospital, Heidelberg

GOODWIN, W. E., M. D., F. A. C. S., Professor of Surgery and Urology, Chief of the Division of Urology, University of California School of Medicine, Los Angeles

GRIFFITH, C. A., M. D., F. A. C. S., Clinical Associate Professor of Surgery, University of Washington School of Medicine, Seattle

GROB, M., Dr., Professor of Pediatric Surgery and Chief, Department of Surgery, Pediatric University Hospital, Zürich

GRÖZINGER, K.-H., Dr., Lecturer, Surgical University Hospital, Heidelberg

GUSBERG, S. B., M. D., F. A. C. S., Professor and Chairman of Obstetrics and Gynecology, Mount Sinai School of Medicine, New York

GÜTGEMANN, A., Dr. med., Professor of Surgery and Director, Surgical University Hospital, Bonn-Venusberg

HALLER, J. A., JR., M. D., F. A. C. S., Robert Garrett Professor of Pediatric Surgery, John Hopkins Hospital and University School of Medicine, Baltimore

HAMMOND, G., M. D., F. A. C. S., Chairman, Orthopaedic Department, Lahey Clinic Foundation, Boston

HAMPERL, H., Prof. Dr., Director of the Department of Pathology, University of Bonn

HARRISON, E. G., M. D., Consultant in Surgical Pathology and Associate Professor of Pathology, Mayo Clinic and Mayo Graduate School of Medicine, Rochester, Minnesota

HEBERER, G., Prof. Dr., Director, Surgical University Hospital, Cologne

HEGEMANN, G., Dr. med., Professor of Surgery and Director, Surgical University Hospital, Erlangen

HENDREN III, W. H., M. D., F. A. C. S., Surgical Chairman, Children's Service of Massachusetts General Hospital, Boston

HUFFMAN, J. W., M. D., F. A. C. S., Professor of Obstetrics and Gynecology, Northwestern University Medical School, Chicago

JOHANSON, B., Dr., Head of the Plastic Unit, Sahlgrenska Hospital and University, Göteborg

KÄSER, O., M. D., Professor of Obstetrics and Gynecology, Woman's Hospital of the University of Frankfurt am Main

KAY, A. W., M. D., F. R. C. S., Professor, University Department of Surgery, Western Infirmary, Glasgow

KERN, G., Dr. med., Professor of Obstetrics and Gynecology Women's Hospital of the University of Cologne

KERR, W. S., JR., M. D., F. A. C. S., Assistant Clinical Professor of Surgery, Harvard Medical School, Boston

KLOSTERHALFEN, H., Dr. med., Director, Urological University Hospital, Hamburg-Eppendorf

KOLIG, G., Dr. med., Instructor in Surgery, Surgical University Hospital, Heidelberg

LECHNER, F., Dr., Associate Surgeon, Hospital of the Right Bank of the Isar College of Science and Technology, Munich

LEVENTHAL, M. L., M. D., F. A. C. S., Clinical Professor of Obstetrics and Gynecology, Michael Reese Hospital, Chicago

LINDER, F., Dr., M. D., F. R. C. S. (Eng. Hon), F. A. C. S. (Hon.), Professor of Surgery and Chairman, Department of Surgery, University of Heidelberg

LONGMIRE, W. P., JR., M. D., F. A. C. S., Professor and Chairman, Department of Surgery, University of California School of Medicine, Los Angeles

LUTZEYER, W., Dr. med., Professor of Urology, Medical School of Rhein-Westfalen College of Science and Technology, Aachen

LYNCH, J. B., M. D., F. A. C. S., Associate Professor of Plastic and Maxillofacial Surgery, University of Texas Medical Branch, Galveston

MAATZ, R., Prof. Dr. med., Medical Director and Chief of Staff, Auguste-Viktoria City Hospital, Berlin-West

MacKENZIE, W. C., M. D., F. R. C. S. (C), F. A. C. S., Professor of Surgery and Dean of Medicine, University of Alberta Faculty of Medicine, Edmonton

MARBERGER, H., M. D., Head of the Department of Urology, Medical School, University Innsbruck, Austria

MATTHES, T., Prof. Dr. med., Specialist in Thoracic Surgery and Acting Director of the Hospital, German Academy of Science, Berlin, DDR

MAURER, G., Prof. Dr., Director, Surgical University Hospitals, Right Bank of the Isar College of Science and Technology, Munich

McKEEVER, F. M., M. D., F. A. C. S., Clinical Professor Emeritus of Orthopaedic Surgery, University of Southern California School of Medicine, Los Angeles

MEILING, R. L., M. D., F. A. C. S., Dean of Ohio State University College of Medicine, Columbus

MERCADIER, M., Dr., Professor of Surgery, University of Paris

MOORE, M., JR., M. D., F. A. C. S., Associate Clinical Professor of Orthopaedic Surgery, University of Tennessee College of Medicine and Chief, Orthopaedic Department, Methodist Hospital, Memphis

MORRIS, G. C., JR., M. D., F. A. C. S., Associate Professor of Surgery, Baylor University College of Medicine, Houston

MORRIS, J. M., M. D., F. A. C. S., Professor of Gynecology, Yale University School of Medicine, New Haven, Connecticut

MÜLLER, M. E., Dr., Professor and Chief, Department of Orthopaedic Surgery, University of Bern, Switzerland

MULLER, W. H., JR., M. D., F. A. C. S., Professor and Chairman, Department of Surgery, University of Virginia Medical Center, Charlottesville

MULLIGAN, W. J., M. D., F. A. C. S., Assistant Clinical Professor in Obstetrics and Gynecology, Boston Hospital for Woman, Parkway Division Formerly Free Hospital for Woman, Boston, Brookline

NAHUM, A. M., M. D., F. A. C. S., Assistant Professor of Surgery, University of California School of Medicine, Los Angeles

NARDI, G. L., M. D., F. A. C. S., Associate Clinical Professor of Surgery, Harvard Medical School and Visiting Surgeon, Massachusetts General Hospital, Boston

NAVRATIL, E., M. D., F. A. C. S. (Hon.), Professor of Obstetrics and Gynecology, Hospital of Obstetrics and Gynecology, University of Graz, Austria

Ross, D. N., M. B., Ch. B., F. R. C. S. (Eng.), Consultant Thoracic Surgeon, Guy's Hospital and the National Heart Hospital, London

Roth, R. B., M. D., F. A. C. S., Chief, Department of Urology, St. Vincent Hospital, Erie, Pennsylvania

Scardino, P. L., M. D., F. A. C. S., Chief of Urology, Memorial Hospital of Chatham County, Savannah Urological Clinic, Savannah, Georgia

Schäfer, H., Dr., Associate Surgeon, Surgical Hospital, Right Bank of the Isar College of Science and Technology, Munich

Schettler, G., Dr., Professor of Internal Medicine, Medical Hospital of Heidelberg University

Schink, W., Dr., Professor of Surgery and Director, Second Surgical University Hospital, Cologne

Schlegel, J. U., M. D., F. A. C. S., Professor and Chairman, Section of Urology, Department of Surgery, Tulane University School of Medicine, New Orleans

Schmid, E., M. D., D. D. S., Chief, Department of Facial and Oral Surgery, St. Mary's Hospital, Stuttgart

Schmitz, W., Dr. med., Lecturer, Surgical University Hospital, Heidelberg

Schneider, R., M. D., Chief of Staff, Grosshöchstetten Hospital, Bern, Switzerland

Schuchardt, K., Dr. med. dent., Professor and Director, Northwest German Oral Hospital, State University Hospital Eppendorf, Hamburg

Schwaiger, M., Dr., Professor of Surgery and Director, Surgical University Hospital of the University of Freiburg (Brsg.)

Scott, H. W., Jr., M. D., F. A. C. S., Professor and Chairman, Department of Surgery, Vanderbilt University School of Medicine, Nashville

Scuderi, C. S., M. D., F. A. C. S., Associate Professor of Orthopaedic Surgery, University of Illinois College of Medicine and Chairman of Orthopaedic Surgery, St. Elizabeth and Columbus Hospitals, Chicago

Shires, G. T., M. D., F. A. C. S., Professor and Chairman, Department of Surgery, University of Texas Southwestern Medical School, Dallas

Skoog, T., M. D., F. A. C. S. (Hon.), Professor of Plastic Surgery, University of Uppsala Faculty of Medicine, Sweden

Smith, M. L., M. D., F. A. C. S., Col., U. S. A., M. C., Surgical Consultant, United States Army, Europe and Seventh Army, Heidelberg

Spence, H. M., M. D., F. A. C. S., Clinical Professor of Urology and Chairman, Division of Urology, University of Texas Southwestern Medical School, Dallas

Spencer, F. C., M. D., F. A. C. S., Professor and Chairman, Department of Surgery, New York University Medical Center, New York

Starr, A., M. D., F. A. C. S., Professor of Surgery and Chief of Cardiopulmonary Surgery, University of Oregon Medical School, Portland

Turner-Warwick, R. T., M. D., F. R. C. S. (Eng.), Chief of Urology, Institute of Urology and the Middlesex Hospital, London

Vollmar, J., Dr., Lecturer, Surgical University Hospital, Heidelberg

Voorhees, A. B., Jr., M. D., F. A. C. S., Associate Professor of Clinical Surgery, Columbia University College of Physicians and Surgeons and Columbia-Presbyterian Medical Center, New York

Vossschulte, K., Professor Dr. med., President, German Surgical Society and Professor of Surgery, Surgical University Hospital, Giessen

Wachsmuth, W., Dr. med., Professor of Surgery and Chairman, Department of Surgery, Surgical University Hospital, Würzburg

Warren, W. D., M. D., F. A. C. S., Professor of Surgery and Dean, University of Miami School of Medicine, Miami

WELCH, C. E., M. D., F. A. C. S., Clinical Professor of Surgery, Harvard Medical School and Visiting Surgeon, Massachusetts General Hospital, Boston

WENZ, W., Dr., Lecturer, Surgical University Hospital, Heidelberg

WILLENEGGER, H., M. D., Professor of Surgery, University of Basle and Head of the Surgical Hospital of Kanton, Liestal, Switzerland

WILSON, J. C., JR., M. D., F. A. C. S., Clinical Professor of Orthopaedic Surgery, University of Southern California School of Medicine and Head, Division of Orthopaedic Surgery, Children's Hospital of Los Angeles

WILSON, P. D., JR., M. D., F. A. C. S., Associate Professor of Orthopaedic Surgery, Cornell University Medical College Hospital for Special Surgery, New York

WITT, A. N., Professor Dr., Director, Orthopaedic Hospital and Policlinic, Free University of Berlin

WYLIE, E. J., M. D., F. A. C. S., Professor of Surgery and Chief of Vascular Surgery, University of California School of Medicine, San Francisco

ZANDER, J., Dr. med., Professor of Obstetrics and Gynecology and Chairman, Department of Obstetrics and Gynecology, University of Heidelberg

ZENKER, R., Dr. M. D., F. A. C. S. (Hon.), Professor of Surgery and Director, Surgical University Hospital, Munich

ZOLLINGER, R. M., M. D., F. A. C. S., Professor and Chairman, Department of Surgery, Ohio State University Medical Center, Columbus

ZUIDEMA, G. D., M. D., F. A. C. S., Professor and Director, Department of Surgery, Johns Hopkins University School of Medicine, Baltimore

ZUKSCHWERDT, L., Dr. med., Professor of Surgery and Director, Surgical University Hospital, Hamburg-Eppendorf

Gynecology

Surgical Treatment of Defects of the Uterovaginal Tract

Josef Zander

According to Antonii de Haen the first attempt of a surgical correction of a congenital absence of vagina was made in 1761 by an unknown surgeon. During this operation where he tried to create an opening between the bladder and rectum, the bladder and the urethra had been perforated. The 24 year old patient died 3 days later. Another attempt had been made about 150 years ago by Dupuytren (1817). [For historical review see Schmid (1956) and Steinmetz (1940).]

Since that time many operative techniques have been reported. They are compiled in Table 1. Larger series of operative construction of an artificial vagina, published in the world literature are summarized in Table 2. It can be estimated that about 1500 cases operated with different techniques have been reported until recently.

The principle of a simple reconstruction of the vagina was used by Wells (1935), Kanter (1935), Wharton (1938) and others (see Table 1). These methods were based on the tendency of the epithelium from the vestible to grow in, and line the vagina if the cavity is kept open. The disadvantages of this method were the slowness with which epithelialization proceeded particularly in the upper part of the created cavity, and its occasional total failure to produce skin. This led frequently to vaginal strictures.

Based on anatomical studies a modification of this method, the boring a double barreled canal, has been reported by Sheares (1960). As a result islands of epithelium of the vestiges of the Müllerian ducts are surfaced and serve a secondary sources of squamous epithelium.

Methods using ileal transplants or rectal transplants were described by Baldwin (1904) and Mori (1910) and by Popoff (1910) and Schubert (1911) respectively. Today they are used only in rare cases. The mortality rates in the preantibiotic period reached 10 to 20% and even more.

More satisfactory results were reported with methods using a portion of the sigmoid colon in the construction of a vagina by Schmid (1956), Shirodkar (1960) and by Alexandrow and Gigovskij (cited by Schmid, 1956) in Russia. Schmid calculated for 311 collected cases of Rostock, Berlin, Moskau and some other places a mortality rate of 1.6%. Using this method a vagina with adequate lubrication and little tendency to contracture can be formed.

Flapp-swinging operations with labial and thigh grafts in different modifications have been also used for the formation of an artificial vagina. Disadvantages were the tendency of the vaginal cavity to contract down-ward, the distortion and deformity of the external genitalia, and finaly the formation of large scars on the thighs.

The transplantation devised by Thiersch was tried by many surgeons and gynecologists. Kirchner and Wagner (1930) used a rubber sponge prothesis covered with a THIERSCH graft. Among the modifications the so called McIndoe-Read technique, first described by McINDOE and BANISTER (1937) is widely used. The graft-covered mould is inserted into the preformed cavity, and a perineal bridge is built beneath it so that it cannot slip out. The mould is left in place for 3 to 6 month and then renewed and replaced by a polythene dilator.

Table 1. *Methods of construction of an artificial vagina*

Method	Authors
Simple reconstruction (Wharton method)	KANTER (1935), WELLS (1935), SCHMIDT-ELMENDORFF (1937), using vernix caseosa, WHARTON (1938, 1940), COUNSELLER (1948), WORD (1951), BARROWS (1957), SHEARES (1960), EVANS (1967), CALI and PRATT (1968)
Fetal membranes (Burger method)	BRINDEAU (1934), BURGER (1937), RUNGE (1951)
Pedunculated grafts (Labial and tigh flaps)	BECK (1900), GRAVES (1921), FRANK and GEIST (1927), DAVIS and CRON (1928), FALLS (1940), BRADY (1945)
Free skin grafts (Kirschner-Wagner or McIndoe-Read method)	ABBE (1898), KIRSCHNER and WAGNER (1930), FLYNN and DUCKET (1936), McINDOE and BANISTER (1938), COUNSELLER (1938), READ (1944), WHARTON (1946), COUNSELLER (1948), BRYAN et al. (1949), McINDOE (1950), THOMPSON et al. (1957), TURUNEN (1957), COUNSELLER and FLOR (1957), JONES (1959), JACKSON (1965), EVANS (1967), CALI and PRATT (1968).
Intestinal transplantation Small intestine (Baldwin-Mori method)	BALDWIN (1904), MORI (1910), BRYAN et al. (1949), COUNSELLER and FLOR (1957)
Rectum (Popoff-Schubert method)	SNEGUIREFF (1904), POPOFF (1910), SCHUBERT (1911, 1933, 1936), SOUSTELLE et al. (1967)
Sigmoid (Schmid method)	SCHMID (1956), SHIRODKAR (1960), COUNSELLER and FLOR (1957)
Formation of large perineum with the inner sides of labia majora	WILLIAMS (1964)
Simple pressure (Frank method)	FRANK (1938), STEINMETZ (1940), HOLMES and WILLIAMS (1940)

According to McINDOE (1950) the most important principles of inlay grafting are:
1. Careful preparation of the cavity,
2. Complete haemostasis and asepsis,
3. Thin split graft in one piece,
4. Continuous (not intermittent) dilatation until the contractile phase is overcome.

JACKSON (1965) described recently 128 cases operated with this technique within a 27 year period in the Chelsea Hospital for Women and in the Middlesex Hospital in London. The results were anatomically satisfactory in 85% of the cases and anatomically unsatisfactory in 5% of the cases. 10% were failures and these included 6 patients with rectal fistulas and 6 patients who refused to finish treatment.

In another recent study CALI and PRATT (1968) reported longterm results of 131 operations with the McIndoe technique within a 46 year period in the Mayo Clinic.

Of 113 traced patients 48 (42%) had some contraction of the vagina or stenosis. Yet 84 (90%) of 93 patients reporting on sexual function expressed satisfaction with function of the organ. There were 30 (22%) complete failures and 31 partial failures of the operative method. The total number of anatomic failures was 46,5% of 131 McIndoe operations.

Table 2. *Larger series of operative construction of an artificial vagina*

	Time period in years	Simple reconstruction	Free skin graft	Bowel transplants	Other methods
Chelsea Hospital for Women and Middlesex Hospital (JACKSON, 1965)	27		128[a]		
Johns Hopkins Hospital (THOMPSON, WHARTON, TeLINDE, 1957)	14		32		
Mayo Clinic (CALI and PRATT, 1968)	46	25	123[b]	19[c]	8
Univ. of Malaya, Singapore (SHEARES, 1960)	5	18			
Univ. of Helsinki (TURUNEN, 1957)	20		47		
Univ.-Frauenklinik Kiel (SMOLKA, 1962)	15	30[d]			
Univ.-Frauenklinik Heidelberg, 1968	26	25[e]	20		
Wayne State Univ. and Univ. of Michigan (EVANS, 1967)		23	87[f]		
Collected cases of Rostock, Berlin and Moskau (SCHMID, 1956)				311[g]	

[a] 63 cases previously reported by McINDOE (1950) and 39 cases reported by McINDOE and SIMMONS (1959) are included in this series.

[b] Cases reported by BRYAN et al. (1949) and COUNSELLER and FLOR (1957) are included in this series.

[c] 13 cases with transplantation of small intestinum and 6 cases with transplantation of sigmoid.

[d] Cases performed with the Burger plastic using fetal membranes are included in this series.

[e] Performed with the Burger plastic using fetal membranes and previously described by RUNGE (1951) and by EBERLE (1959)

[f] 71 cases previously reported by MILLER et al. (1945) and by MILLER and STOUT (1957) are included in this series.

[g] Transplantation of sigmoid.

TURUNEN (1957) reported the results of 47 operations performed within a 20 year period in the Department of Obstetrics and Gynecology of the University of Helsinki using the Thiersch graft technique. Satisfactory results were obtained in 74% of the patients. According to a recent summary by EVANS (1967) of 110 cases operated in the Departments of Obstetrics and Gynecology of the Wayne State University and the University of Michigan a good result was achieved in 75% of the cases. The fistula rate was about 5%.

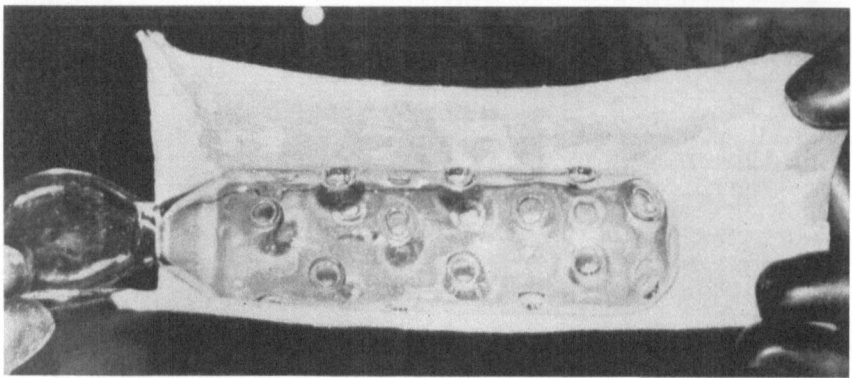

Fig. 1. The glass mould on the free skin graft. The small holes allow the irrigation of the vagina during the postoperative days

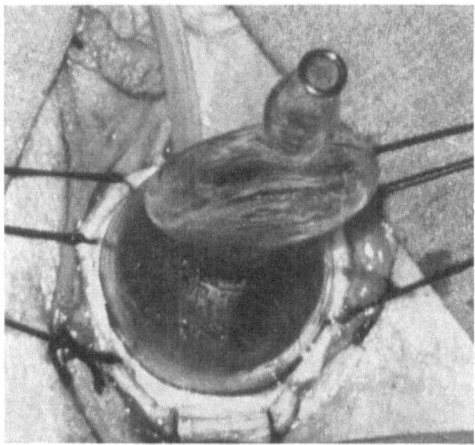

Fig. 2. The graft covered glass mould is inserted into the preformed cavity

At the Department of Obstetrics and Gynecology of the University of Heidelberg within a 26 year period 45 cases were operated. Until some years ago the so called Burger plastic (1937) using fetal membranes and first described by BRINDEAU (1934) has been used. The long-time results with this method were satisfactory in 64% of the cases (RUNGE, 1951; EBERLE, 1959). Postoperative rectovaginal fistulas were observed in two cases. Since 1964 a free skin graft method has been the method of choice.

In the preparation of the cavity and the thin split graft we follow the principles of McINDOE (1950) as described above. A glass mould with small holes is used which allows the irrigation of the vagina during the postoperative days (Figs. 1 and 2). It is removed between the 12th and 14th day after the operation and immediately replaced by a Plexi glass mould. This prothesis as a general rule is worn at least for a period of 2 years continuously.

Selection of patients. Some authors believe that only those women who are married, or who are engaged should be accepted for surgical treatment. I can not agree with this general statement. An individual decision seems to be necessary in every case after careful psychologic exploration of the personality. In some cases the knowledge of the absence of the vagina can result in marked feeling of inferiority and this again can prevent a more intimate contact with the male sex. The patient can be protected against the premature contraction of the artificial vagina by the mould. Regular sexual intercourse is therefore not a factor necessary in the prevention of contractions.

The basal body temperature should be measured in every patient before operation. Today laparotomy is not indicated if biphasic temperatures are registrated and hematometra can be excluded.

Absence of ovarian function can not be regarded as a contraindication against the formation of an artificial vagina. However the genetic and endocrine diagnosis should be made before the operation is done.

It is well known, that abnormalities of the urinary tract (pelvic kidney, solitary kidney, horseshoe kidney, duplication of the ureters or renal pelvis) are frequently associated with congenital absence of the vagina. Urologic investigation including pyelogram is therefore essential in every patient before operation.

The mould. All sorts of material have been used to form the mould. We prefer an open glass mould with small holes for drainage which allows to irrigate the vagina after the operation. It is hold with a T-bandage. A few days before the patient is dismissed from the hospital she receives a plexi glass mould as long-time prothesis. This mould is formed according to the individual form of the vagina. The long-time mould is considered to be good, if after a while the women does not feel it any more.

Many different shapes have been designed for the mould. Mostly the cylindrical form is prefered. A remarkable modification has been recently described by STABLER (1966). Since normally at rest the front and back walls of the vagina are in contact, and only during coitus is the cylindrical form produced, a flattened form of mould was designed which maintains the physiological shape of the vagina during the whole of the postoperative period. This form may have indeed some advantages over the usual cylindrical shaped prothesis.

Special problems are involved in cases with a functional uterus, hematometra and congenital absence of the vagina, or vagina and cervix. FIKENTSCHER and SEMM (1966) have described a combined vaginal-intrauterine prothesis for those cases. We made successful use of this prothesis in a 13 year old girl 2 years ago. The patient is menstruating regularly. Today exstirpation of a functioning uterus should be avoided. Pregnancies and deliveries have been reported in many cases after the construction of an artificial vagina in cases where the uterus was functioning (WAGNER, 1923, 1927; WHITTMORE, 1942; READ, 1944; BAER, 1947; BAER and DE COSTA, 1947; POTOTSCHNIG, 1949; FAUVET, 1952; SOLOMONS, 1956; EVANS, 1967).

The contractile phase. According to McINDOE the contractile phase is common to all forms of free grafted skin. Inlay grafts, which line concave surfaces, suffer from this phase more severely than any other type of free graft. The time period of the contractile phase seems to be different from case to case. During the contractile phase remarkable contraction of the upper third of the artificial vagina can occur if the prothesis is only removed for a night or a few days. Carefully controlled continuous dilatation is essential during the entire phase until healing and resolution are complete, and the tendency to contract has entirely ceased. CALI and PRATT recently reported that in 123 patients a vaginal mould was necessary for an average of about 2 years. In several instances moulds were utilized for more than 15 years. The early removal of the mould is particularly dangerous if epithelialization of the vagina is not complete. Too early removal of the mould is one of the major reasons for unsatisfactory results or failures. It is an advantage of the bowel methods that contraction seem to occur only to a minor extent.

Complications. Among the postoperative complications in the free graft techniques, vaginal and urinary infections have been observed primerally. Vaginal infections can prevent the healing of the graft. We have the impression that spong rubber moulds may favour vaginal infections. Since we irrigated the vagina postoperatively through the mould, vaginal infections were not observed any more. Urine cultures should be carried out routinely. Prophylactic use of antibiotics is necessary.

Rectovaginal, vesicovaginal and urethrovaginal fistulas can occur occasionally as serious complication during or after the operation. Rectovaginal fistulas have been more often observed than vesicovaginal fistulas, even several months after the operation. In some cases they healed spontaneously. Using the McIndoe technique, where the mould is left continuously in place for several months it has been observed that, in several cases the mould was passed per rectum. In repeated operations with extensive formation of scars the risk of damage of the rectum or bladder is significantly higher than in the first operation.

Other complications are haemorrhages, and seldom deep vein thrombosis.

The formation of vaginal granulation is a characteristic complication of the free skin graft methods. The granulation tissue is formed in areas where the graft has not survived. The granulation tissue is often found in the vault of the vagina. The granulation prevents epithelialization of this area and it is essential that these granulations be removed by currettage or cautery. In some cases a second graft is necessary. Since most of the patients have a ovulatory menstrual cycle, additional treatment with estrogens is not necessary. We have the impression that local treatment with estrogen ointment even stimulates the growth of granulation tissue.

References

ABBE, R.: Med. Rec. (N.Y.) **54**, 836 (1898).
ALEXANDROW, M. S.: Cited by H. H. SCHMID, Scheidenbildung aus dem S-förmigen Dickdarm. Jena: VEB Gustav Fischer 1956.
BALDWIN, J. F.: Ann. Surg **40**, 398 (1904).
BAER, J. L.: J. Mt Sinai Hosp. **14**, 244 (1947).
—, and J. DeCosta: Amer. J. Obstet. Gynec. **54**, 696 (1947).
BARROWS, D. N.: Amer. J. Obstet. Gynec. **73**, 609 (1957).
BECK, C.: Ann. Surg. **32**, 572 (1900).
BRADY, L.: Ann. Surg. **121**, 518 (1945).
BRINDEAU, A.: Gynéc. et Obstét. **29**, 885 (1934).
BRYAN, A. L., I. A. NIGRO, and V. S. COUNSELLER: Surg. Gynec. Obstet. **88**, 79 (1949).
BURGER, K.: Zbl. Gynäc. **61**, 2437 (1937).
CALI, R. W., and J. H. PRATT: Amer. J. Obstet. Gynec. **100**, 752 (1968).
COUNSELLER, V. S.: Amer. J. Obstet. Gynec. **36**, 632 (1938).
— J. Amer. med. Ass. **136**, 861 (1948).
—, and F. S. FLOR: Surg. Clin. N. Amer. **37**, 1107 (1957).

DAVIS, C. H., and R. S. CRON: Amer. J. Obstet. Gynec. **15**, 196 (1928).

DEHAEN, A.: Cit. by B. WORD. Sth. med. J. (Bgham. Ala.) **44**, 375 (1951).

EBERLE, H.: Medizinische **8**, 332 (1959).

EVANS, T. N.: Amer. J. Obstet. Gynec. **99**, 944 (1967).

FALLS, F. H.: Amer. J. Obstet. Gynec. **40**, 906 (1940).

FAUVET, E.: Geburtsh. u. Frauenheilk. **12**, 897 (1952).

FIKENTSCHER, R., u. K. SEMM: Geburtsh. u. Frauenheilk. **26**, 132 (1966).

FLYNN, C. W., and J. W. DUCKET: Surg. Gynec. Obstet. **62**, 753 (1936).

FRANK, R. T.: Amer. J. Obstet. Gynec. **35**, 1053 (1938).

—, and S. H. GEIST: Amer. J. Obstet. Gynec. **14**, 712 (1927).

GIGOWSKIJ, E. E.: Cited by H. H. SCHMID, Scheidenbildung aus dem S-förmigen Dickdarm. Jena: VEB Gustav Fischer 1956.

GRAVES, W. P.: Surg. Clin. N. Amer. **1**, 611 (1921).

HOLMES, W. R., and G. A. WILLIAMS: Amer. J. Obstet. Gynec. **39**, 145 (1940).

JACKSON, J.: J. Obstet. Gynaec. Brit. Cwlth **72**, 336 (1965).

JONES, H. W.: Clin. Obstet. Gynec. **2**, 1053 (1959).

KANTER, A. E.: Amer. J. Surg. **30**, 314 (1935).

KIRSCHNER, M., and G. A. WAGNER: Zbl. Gynäk. **43**, 2690 (1930).

McINDOE, A. H.: Brit. J. plast. Surg. **2**, 254 (1950).

—, and J. B. BANISTER: J. Obstet. Gynaec. Brit. Emp. **45**, 490 (1938).

—, and C. A. SIMMONS: Proc. roy. Soc. Med. **52**, 952 (1959).

MILLER, N. F., and W. STOUT: Obstet. and Gynec. **9**, 48 (1957).

—, J. R. WILLSON, and J. COLLINS: Amer. J. Obstet. Gynec. **50**, 735 (1945).

MORI, M.: Zbl. Gynäk. **33**, 172 (1909); **34**, 11 (1910).

POPOFF, D. D.: Russk. Vrach. St. Petersb. **60**, 1512 (1910); Cited by McINDOE, Brit. J. plast. Surg. **2**, 254 (1950).

POTOTSCHNIG, G.: Zbl. Gynäk. **71**, 792 (1949).

READ, C. D.: Irish J. med. Sci. **6**, 52 (1944).

RUNGE, H.: Zbl. Gynäk. **73**, 599 (1951).

SCHMID, H. H.: Die Scheidenbildung aus dem S-förmigen Dickdarm. Jena: VEB Gustav Fischer 1956.

SCHMIDT-ELMENDORFF, H. R.: Zbl. Gynäk. **45**, 2602 (1937).

SCHUBERT, G.: Ber. ges. Gynäk. Geburtsh. **23**, 241 (1933).

— Die künstliche Scheidenbildung aus dem Mastdarm nach SCHUBERT. Stuttgart: Enke 1936.

— Zbl. Gynäk. **35**, 1017 (1911).

SHEARES, B. H.: J. Obstet. Gynaec. Brit. Emp. **67**, 24 (1960).

SHIRODKAR, V. N.: Contributions to Obstet. and Gynec. Edinburgh: E. and S. Livingstone Ltd. 1960.

SMOLKA, H.: Geburtsh. u. Frauenheilk. **22**, 1187 (1962).

SNEGUIREFF, W. F.: Zbl. Gynäk. **28**, 772 (1904).

SOLOMONS, E.: Obstet. and Gynec. **7**, 329 (1956).

SOUSTELLE, J., H. VILLIERS et P. VUILLARD: Traitement chirurgical de l'aplasie vaginale. Lyon: S.I.M.E.P. Editions 1967.

STABLER, F.: J. Obstet. Gynaec. Brit. Cwlth **73**, 463 (1966).

STEINMETZ, E. P.: West. J. Surg. **48**, 169 (1940).

THOMPSON, J. D., L. R. WHARTON, and R. W. TELINDE: Amer. J. Obstet. Gynec. **74**, 397 (1957).

TURUNEN, A.: Ann. Chir. Gynaec. Fenn. **46**, 121 (1957).

—, and C. E. UNNÉRUS: Acta obstet. gynec. scand. **46**, 99 (1967).

WAGNER, G. A.: Arch. Gynäk. **120**, 136 (1923).

— Zbl. Gynäk. **51**, 1302 (1927).

WELLS, W. F.: Amer. J. Surg. **29**, 253 (1935).

WHARTON, L. R.: Ann. Surg. **107**, 842 (1938).

— Ann. Surg. **111**, 1010 (1940).

— Amer. J. Obstet. Gynec. **51**, 866 (1946).

WHITTMORE, W. S.: Amer. J. Obstet. Gynec. **44**, 516 (1942).

WILLIAMS, E. A.: J. Obstet. Gynaec. Brit. Cwlth **71**, 511 (1964).

WORD, B.: Sth. Med. J. (Bgham. Ala.) **44**, 375 (1951).

Polycystic Ovarian Disease

Michael L. Leventhal

Polycystic ovarian disease is an entity in which the anovulatory ovary can be converted into an ovulatory one. Wedge resection of the ovaries, often producing a dramatic and irreversible return of hormonal homeostasis, has been the treatment of choice for many years. First performed in 1895, wedge resection of the ovaries was frequently done in the first part of this century for a wide spectrum of menstrual disorders with varying results. In 1935 Stein and Leventhal brought some order out of chaos by defining a syndrome of polycystic ovaries in which wedge resection, in properly selected cases, was very successful. Since 1950 their results have been confirmed by many observers throughout the world.

Concomitant with the widespread use of wedge resection, other modalities of treatment began to appear and to challenge the surgical approach in the treatment of polycystic ovaries. The ability of some types of polycystic ovary to respond to medications that restore a normal hypothalamo-pituitary-ovarian relationship, even though temporarily, is evidence of the dysfunctional nature of the disease. However, the establishment of prolonged normal function by wedge resection following failure of medical treatment lends support to the view that an organic component (grossly thickened capsules) may have to be removed before proper ovulation can be restored in some patients. It is perhaps these cases, rare in occurrence, which comprise the segment in the broad spectrum of anovulation known as the Stein-Leventhal syndrome.

The important non-surgical modalities in the treatment of polycystic ovarian disease include corticosteroids, clomiphene citrate, human pituitary gonadotropin (HPG) and human menopausal gonadotropin (HMG). Thus, a discussion of the surgical treatment of polycystic ovaries must attempt a comparison of the results of wedge resection with the results of medical treatment.

Corticosteroids

The polycystic ovaries typical of the Stein-Leventhal syndrome have been shown to be an important source of abnormal androgen, producing an increase of plasma testosterone levels. Androgens from this ovarian source contribute little towards an increment of total urinary 17-ketosteroids and are usually associated with normal or, at most, slightly elevated values. They are not however, responsive to corticosteroid suppressive therapy. If regular menstruation does follow suppressive therapy, it is likely that the anovulation is due to a type of mild postpubertal or borderline adrenocortical syndrome. Patients with this condition are indistinguishable clinically from patients with the Stein-Leventhal syndrome. Enlarged polycystic ovaries are present in about 50% of these patients but wedge resection notoriously fails; and, it is in these failures that subsequent corticosteroid therapy may be effective. When the typical polycystic ovary is associated with secondarily induced adrenocortical hyperfunction, corticosteroids may induce ovulation. However, after 1 or 2 menstrual periods, amenorrhea usually recurs in spite of continued therapy. Such patients then often respond to wedge resection. Markedly increased excretion of 17-ketosteroids, as a rule, eliminates the ovary as the source of abnormal androgen and should direct attention to the adrenal gland itself.

Gonadotropins

Anovulatory patients with low urinary gonadotropins and little or no detectable estrogen activity have the worst prognosis for the return of homeostatic hormonal activity, but are best treated with pituitary gonadotropins in conjunction with human chorionic gonadotropin (HCG). Even though this situation does not exist with typical polycystic ovaries (in which urinary gonadotropins are normal and there is good evidence of endogenous estrogen activity), gonadotropins have been used with some success in patients with the syndrome as well as in patients with other types of anovulation, Pergonal (HMG) is the one most available for clinical use. Gonadotropin prepared from postmortem human pituitaries, used in a few select research centers, is not available commercially for clinical studies. The biologic activity of the two is predominantly that of FSH, and is identical. At the present time there is difficulty in assaying the concentration of FSH and LH in human gonadotropin, and although proper dosage schedules have not been definitely determined, excellent results have been obtained by TAYMOR et al. (1967) and others by monitoring the gonadotropin dose with daily estrogen excretion levels. Gonadotropins have been used successfully after clomiphene and wedge resection failures in some patients in whom the anovulation was based on a presumed diagnosis of the Stein-Leventhal syndrome. These are probably patients who have low estrogen secretion as manifested by vaginal smear and atrophic endometrium, and perhaps should have been treated by gonadotropins initially. They require human pituitary gonadotropins plus sequential HCG in order to achieve follicular maturation and ovulation. In retrospect they should not have been included in the category of the syndrome.

Patients with the syndrome should be treated with gonadotropins, if at all, only with great care and experience and only after failure of clomiphene, clomiphene-HCG and wedge resection. The possibility of dangerous overstimulation of the extremely responsive follicles in the polycystic ovary is real, requiring frequent pelvic examinations and careful titering of the gonadotropin dose to the patient's level of total estrogen. As with clomiphene, the number of pregnancies is relatively low compared to the high percentage of apparent ovulations. GEMZELL reported an 80% ovulation rate, a 40% pregnancy rate of which 44% were multiple, and an abortion rate of 25% in his series of patients with secondary amenorrhea treated with HPG. TAYMOR et al. (1967), using HMG in a selected group of patients who failed to ovulate with clomiphene, reported a 63% pregnancy rate in 24 amenorrheic patients. In a larger series of cases of anovulation treated with HMG, he reported an overall ovulation rate of 72% and a pregnancy rate of 26%. The abortion rate was 25% and there were only 10% multiple pregnancies compared to 44% reported with HPG. It is obvious that even ready availability of human gonadotropins, which is not likely, will not make the more effective and safer modalities of treatment of polycystic ovaries, such as clomiphene and wedge resection, obsolete.

Clomiphene Citrate

It has been well established that clomiphene citrate is capable of inducing ovulation in a wide spectrum of menstrual disturbances associated with anovulation. Included in the spectrum is a segment occupied by an endocrine disturbance characterized by *enlarged* ovaries, with varying degrees of *thickening of the capsule* and with small subcapsular cysts. These ovaries may produce abnormal amounts of androgen. When these patients exhibit urinary gonadotropins in the normal range, show evidence of endogenous estrogen activity, and have essentially normal 17-ketosteroids, a therapeutic course of clomiphene, if otherwise not contraindicated, is very often rewarding in inducing ovulation. However, since pregnancy is the only irrefutable evidence of ovulation, the results of treatment of anovulation by any modality is best analyzed from the standpoint of the pregnancy rate. In a group of 24 patients with the Stein-Leventhal syndrome, COHEN reported an 80% ovulation rate but only 35% became pregnant. 6 of the patients were considered to be clomiphene failures, and 5 of these conceived promptly following subsequent wedge resection. SCOMMEGNA treated 18 patients with a presumed diagnosis of Stein-Leventhal syndrome, of whom 17 ovulated (90%). Pregnancy was desired in 11 of the ovulators, and of these only 4 or 36% conceived. 1 patient failed to respond to clomiphene, but conceived promptly following wedge resection. According to KISTNER (1965) who analyzed large numbers of reports, about 75% of infertile polycystic ovary syndrome patients will respond to clomiphene with ovulation, but only 40 to 45% will conceive. Thus there appears to be a discrepancy between the ovulatory rate and the expected number of pregnancies.

Why is there such a discrepancy? It should first be acknowledged that such a difference could be more apparent than real. There are no reports in which clomiphene-induced and normal pregnancy rates are compared with regard to length of exposure while ovulating, patient's age, and coital frequency. In many, only infrequent mention is made of investigation of male factors. However, assuming that this discrepancy *is* a real one, is it possible to postulate a reason on an ovarian basis? It is well known that the tunica albuginea in the typical polycystic ovary is invariably thickened, stands out in marked contrast to the underlying stroma, and contains no primordial follicles. The thick fibrous capsule is due to hyperplasia and hypertrophy of collagen fibers, which may increase the diameter of the layer 2 to 6 fold. A study of some wedges from enlarged ovaries due to overstimulation with clomiphene revealed luteinization of cystic follicles and corpora lutea under a thickened capsule. Progesterone secreted from these structures would produce clinical and laboratory findings typical of ovulation without the occurrence of external ovulation. In one ovary we have observed rupture of an ovum from a mature follicle into an adjacent cystic follicle, under a thickened tunic. This patient became pregnant after wedge resection and continued to have regular ovulatory cycles. PEREZ-PELAEZ described a patient who had evidence of ovulation after extensive treatment with clomiphene. Resected wedges from her ovaries revealed several corpora lutea inside the parenchyma of the ovaries. There is evidence to suggest that patients with *prolonged* amenorrhea associated with *large* ovaries are less likely to become pregnant following clomiphene therapy than patients with the syndrome of shorter duration and perhaps smaller ovaries. FERRIMAN et al., in comparing *ovulatory response* in relation to *ovarian size* showed that patients with large polycystic ovaries fare better than those with normal sized ovaries. However, their conception rate was lower. He stated that "perhaps the thickened capsules of the polycystic ovaries interfere with the release of ova; or, the increased production of androgen by these ovaries impairs nidation". He also showed that ovulatory response was better when the estrogen excretion level exceeded 21 μg/24 h. This correlates well with the better response obtained in patients with marked proliferative or hyperplastic endometrium.

Is it possible that when the typical polycystic ovary is treated medically, the extremely thickened capsule prevents external ovulation? It would be pertinent to the above proposal to know whether patients becoming pregnant on clomiphene have a thin capsule and if the failures have a thick one. Perhaps the latter are the ones that require wedge resection. Since it is impossible to know this before surgery, it is logical that clomiphene should be tried as the initial form of therapy.

Cases meeting all the criteria for the Stein-Leventhal syndrome are rare. STEIN (1966) collected 108 cases in 35 years of active practice. INGERSOLL collected only 21 cases of typical polycystic ovaries (with ovarian enlargement of 2 to 5 times) in 27 years. In the widely quoted article by GOLDZIEHER and AXELROD, close scrutiny of the large numbers of cases of presumed Stein-Leventhal syndrome that they collected from the literature makes it obvious that the inclusion of many reported cases into the syndrome is not substantiated.

Wedge Resection of the Ovaries

That favorable results are obtained with wedge resection in patients with the typical Stein-Leventhal syndrome is indisputable. It is possible that infertile patients with prolonged amenorrhea, who have enlarged ovaries with marked capsular thickening are more likely to become pregnant following wedge resection than by medical treatment. It is my impression from personal experience that this is so. It is important to rule out all other causes of anovulation and to filter out these select cases for surgical treatment. This may be difficult because the etiology in a majority of these patients is often obscure. It would therefore be prudent to treat all patients whose anovulation appears to be the basis of their infertility and who show evidence of adequate endogenous estrogen, initially with clomiphene citrate. If such a course fails to induce ovulation within no less than 6 months, then clomiphene plus sequential HCG should be used. This combination has been shown to increase the ovulation percentage by 20% over clomiphene alone, and also to increase the pregnancy rate. Following failure with this, wedge resection may produce a beneficial result. Since most patients with the Stein-Leventhal syndrome exhibit an apparent ovulatory response to clomiphene (80 to 90%), but only 40 to 50% of these become pregnant, the surgical treatment of polycystic ovaries must remain an important modality of treatment. STEIN (1964) reported a pregnancy rate as high as 85% in his private series. Pregnancy rates following wedge resection vary widely in reported series. Having reviewed the literature, I feel that a higher pregnancy rate than the 40 to 50% reported for clomiphene might have been obtained by a more careful selection of cases for wedge resection. The restoration of ovulation following wedge resection may be permanent, as compared to the temporary restoration of function following clomiphene treatment, which most often is limited to the treatment cycle. One potential complication of wedge resection is the formation of peritubal and periovarian adhesions as reported by KISTNER (1968). If it occurs, and its occurrence obviously has to do with surgical technique as well as host response, it may in itself prevent pregnancy even though ovulation is established.

The polycystic ovary syndrome should be treated at all ages when accurately diagnosed. In the young unmarried patients, including late teen-agers, it is not necessary to establish ovulatory cycles. If hirsuitism is a disturbing symptom, suppression of the ovary by cyclic therapy with estrogen-progestin combinations is valuable in reducing the abnormal androgen production. Cyclic progesterone may also be used. It will cause regular monthly bleedings and oppose the prolonged uninterrupted estrogen stimulation of the endometrium, thus preventing hyperplastic and anaplastic changes. Wedge resection may be rarely indicated in the young unmarried woman who has developed a neurosis about her abnormal menstrual function and defeminization. If medical therapy is unsuccessful in married infertile women with the syndrome, wedge resection may be effective. Long term results from wedge resection seem to continue to justify its place in the treatment of the polycystic ovary syndrome. Correct diagnosis and proper selection of cases for surgery is often a difficult task. The ultimate treatment of the syndrome will probably have to await an exact delineation of the basic metabolic defect.

References

COHEN, M. R.: Fertil. and Steril. 17, 765 (1966).
FERRIMAN, D., A. W. PURDIE, and M. CORNS: Brit. med. J. 4, 444 (1967).
GEMZELL, C.: Clin. Obstet. Gynec. 10, 401 (1967).
GOLDZIEHER, J. W., and L. R. AXELROD: Fert. and Steril. 14, 631 (1963).
INGERSOLL, F. M.: Some anovulation still needs surgery. Obstet. Gynec. digest. 1968.
KISTNER, R. W.: Obstet. gynec. Surv. 20, 873 (1965).
— Peri-tubal and peri-ovarian adhesions subsequent to wedge resection of the ovaries. Presented at the annual meeting of the American Fertility Society, March 29, 1968. Fertil. and Steril. (in press).
PEREZ-PELAEZ, M.: Personal communication.
SCOMMEGNA, A.: Investigator's report on clomiphene. Wm. S. Merrill Co., Cincinnati, Ohio. Personal communication.
STEIN, I. F.: West. J. Surg. 78, 237 (1964).
— In: Ovulation, ed. by R. B. GREENBLATT. Philadelphia: J. B. Lippincott Co. 1966.
—, and M. L. LEVENTHAL: Amer. J. Obstet. Gynec. 29, 181 (1935).
TAYMOR, M. L.: Clin. Obstet. Gynec. 10, 685 (1967).
—, S. H. STURGIS, D. P. GOLDSTEIN, and B. LIEBERMAN: Fertil. and Steril. 18, 181 (1967).

The Role of Fallopian Tubes in Physiology of Conception

WILLIAM J. MULLIGAN

Proper assessment of the role of the Fallopian tubes in physiology of conception requires much more than the time allotted me. It is as though one were compressing a book into a page, and, I, perforce, may dwell only on the highlights with proper consideration of the dynamic and complex role of the oviduct in transport, nuture and the consummation of the mechanism of fertility.

The adult human Fallopian tube is 8 to 15 cm in length and is divided into four zones.

1. An intramural portion actually in the wall of the uterine fundus.

2. The isthmus — about 3 cm in length with lumen averaging 300 micra in diameter and lying distal to the fundus uteri.

3. The ampulla — averaging 7 cm in length with gradually increasing lumenal diameter up to 2 cm at the distal end.

4. The infundibulum, consisting of numerous longitudinal folds of mucous membranes subdividing an ever increasing diameter and terminating in the fimbrial ostium.

The inner mucosa varies from a simple pattern at the isthmus to the longitudinal folds of the ampulla. The projections of mucous membranes at the ampulla float freely in one lumen under normal conditions.

In accordance with the parameso-nephric system, the mucosal cells exhibit varying patterns of activity. The columnar epithelial cells are in part ciliated with the prevailing current directed toward the uterus. Numerous secretory cells are recognized and a "peg-like" supporting cell is present. Even though numerous extensive investigations have been carried out, one may only conclude that the various ciliated and secretory cells are most important in the transport and sustenance of the fertilized ovum.

In passing, it may be noted that the so-called lamina propria of the tube is almost identical in appearance and in cyclic variations with endometrial stroma.

During the growth of the follicle and subsequent rupture, estrogen and progesterone, in ever varying proportions appear to sensitize the entire oviduct to ideally affect maximum fertility. In optimum circumstances the egg or eggs should be quickly transferred to ampulla and subsequent fertilization. BLANDAU has shown this effective mechanism in the rat in a brilliant cinema production of the closed ovisac. Man, the less efficient breeder, presents the end of the oviduct as an open funnel.

We are indebted to WESTMAN for original observations regarding ovum transfer. These observations have been confirmed by many of us through culdoscopy and laparotomy at the time of ovulation. At the time of ovulation approaches the fimbriae contract at an ever increasing rate. The ovary is drawn into a recess in the posterior aspect of the broad ligament. The tubo-ovarian ligament is shortened, bringing the ostium into a position embracing the ovary. Thus a physiologic ovisac is created, and in the absence of pathologic disturbances, the juxta-position facilitates the pick-up mechanism of the tubal ostium.

The ciliary mechanism of the tube sustains a steady stream of fluid from the abdominal cavity to cervix and vagina. This, then, is an initiating factor in transport of the egg into the potentially fertilizing atmosphere of the infundibulum.

Tubal musculature consists of a central circular layer, and an outer-longitudinal layer interspersed with the musculature of serosal vessels and the typical pattern of the isthmus in which inner longitudinal bundles are not clearly defined. As may be expected, the tubo-ovarian ligament exhibits muscular layers beneath the peritoneum. This pattern contributes, of course, to the previously described pick-up mechanism.

According to RADECKI, amular contractions occur without propagation along the tube, and in the gestational tube afford a segmental "to and fro movement" of intratubal contents — thus more or less recapitulating smooth muscle activity in the intestinal tract.

All mammals, according to HARTMAN, require the same time for transport of eggs from ovary to uterus, namely, 3.5 to 4 days. One simple explanation as demonstrated by CHANG, is that this delay affords maturation of eggs and implantation of the fertilized egg into the properly prepared endometrium.

Apparently, as has so brilliantly been demonstrated by Blandau's photography, peristaltic and segmental muscular contractions of the tube results in the egg being rolled back and forth in a single loop for some time and apparently demonstrating peristaltic reaction complexes to ovum sized particles.

Influences on peristalsis are mainly estrogens and progesterone. Estrogen apparently increases the rate, tonus and amplitude of tubal contractions. Most observers agree that the pattern of contractions is modified by progesterone. The role of pituitary extracts, epinephrine, and the prostaglandins has not been properly assessed. But it is increasingly evident from adequate research that priming of the tube with estrogen, as has been demonstrated in the endometrial pattern, is an essential initial step, perhaps providing the "locking mechanism" attributed to the isthmic segment and insuring the release eventually of a maturated ovum available for implantation. Indeed the response of the tubal isthmus and that of the cervical isthmus, under the influence of estrogen and progesterone during pregnancy, invite the prospectus that these are special target tissues, apparently histologically identical with adjacent tissues but possessing unique characteristic response. Perhaps in the presence of adequate estrogen-progesterone balance on the isthmic target tissue, the isthmic block opens and the mature ovum enters the endometrial cavity to seek its destiny.

Roentgenographic and Other Techniques in the Diagnosis of Uterotubal Factors in Sterility and Infertility*

JOHN W. HUFFMAN

WILLIAM ROENTGEN of Würzburg, discoverer of the X-ray, paved the way for those who subsequently developed hysterosalpingographic techniques. LUDLOW (1909) reported calcified fibromyomata of the uterus which had been diagnosed roentgenologically. The first hysterosalpingogram was obtained by RINDFLEISCH (1910) who filled the uterine cavity with a barium paste and then made a roentgenogram which demonstrated the endometrial cavity and the left tube. RUBIN (1914) and CAREY (1914) pioneered in the evolution of uterosalpingography. HEUSER (1925) and STEIN and ARENS (1927) demonstrated the value of hysterosalpingography combined with pneumoperitoneum. It is fitting that we should acknowledge the help which these and many other investigators have given us.

The determination of tubal patency by insufflation, salpingoroentgenography or perfusion is an indispensable part of most infertility studies. In addition, the clinician seeks to determine, when possible, whether there are partial obstructions of the tubes by intratubal disease or extratubal factors and whether there are functional disturbances in tubal motility.

The diagnosis of tubal obstructions by uterotubal insufflation was first made by RUBIN in 1920. His work gave impetus to the interest in infertility which has continued to the present. The investigations of SIEGLER of New York have added immensely to the practical application of uterosalpingography.

The relative merits of insufflation and hysterosalpingography are sometimes debated. Actually, they supplement each other. Insufflation is simpler because it requires relatively inexpensive equipment, can be done in the clinic and is attended by minimal hazards when carbon dioxide is used. It is hoped that air insufflation with its hazard of embolism will soon be abandoned. A kymograph used in conjunction with insufflation will record tubal spasm not easily recorded by hysterosalpingography.

Hysterosalpingography, on the other hand, gives visual evidence of many tubal disorders in addition to obstruction which are related to infertility and sterility. By

* From the Department of Obstetrics and Gynecology, Northwestern University Medical School and the Department of Obstetrics and Gynecology, Passavant Memorial Hospital, Chicago, Illinois.

means of hysterosalpingography it is possible to diagnose tubal diverticula (Fig. 1), tubal tuberculosis, partial tubal occlusion and certain tubal anomalies. Again, it is hoped that rapidly absorbing, non-irritating media, which do not produce foreign body reactions, will soon completely replace oily preparations in the performance of hysterosalpingography.

Inasmuch as tubal spasm may create a false impression of tubal occlusion on either hysterosalpingography or insufflation it is advisable to repeat either or both procedures when there is unexplained tubal blockage.

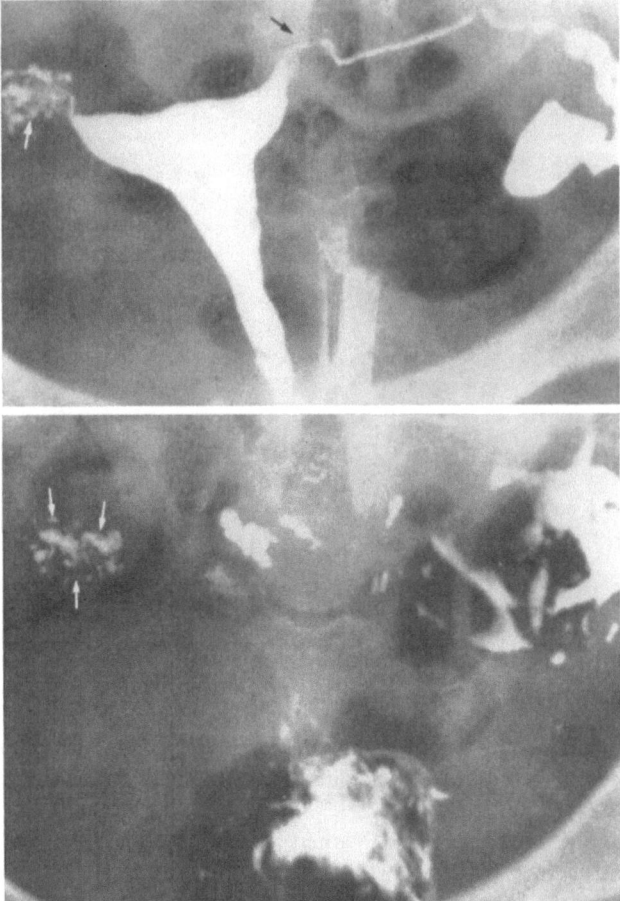

Fig. 1. *Top*, Trabeculation is present in left tubal isthmus (white arrow) with slight, similar changes in the right tube (black arrow). *Bottom*, In a delayed film, taken 1 h later, the medium persists in extraluminal channels (arrows). From SIEGLER, A.: *Hysterosalpingography*. New York: Hoeber Medical Division, Harper and Row, Publishers 1968

There is little doubt that 8 or 16 mm cineuterosalpingography would be a valuable tool for the diagnostician. Cineroentgenography has been of great help in the study of other areas of the body and has been used a few times in the diagnosis of infertility. However, the amount of radiation the ovaries receive during the process of making even a short film is large enough to make its application undesirable. Instead, the uterus and tubes are studied fluoroscopically during the injection of the media and serial films, exposed at significant times, are able to satisfactorily identify abnormalities of uterine and tubal structure and the location of tubal stenoses or obstructions.

It is a moot question whether or not the conceptus is nourished by the tubal secretions. It is known that the tubal mucosa does elaborate monosaccharides during the period the fertilized egg is in the tube. At present we know of no way to evaluate this physiologic component of the reproductive process.

I will not discuss tubal perfusion because I note that Dr. FIKENTSCHER is going to talk about that subject.

Abnormalities of the uterine corpus which interfere with conception are rare. They are much more likely to prevent nidation or to cause abortion. Lesser degrees of uterine growth failure with hypoplasia or persistence of an adolescent cervicocorporeal structural relationship are encountered in infertile women but they are,

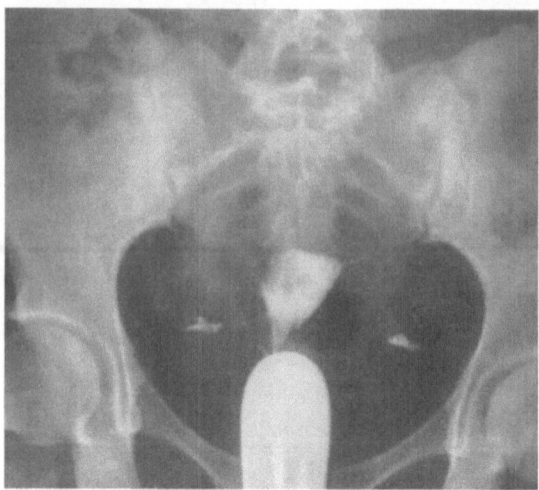

Fig. 2. Hysterogram demonstrates an oval defect in the corpus. A submucus myoma was found at hysterotomy. The patient had had hypermenorrhea and had been infertile for 6 years. Myomectomy was followed by two normal pregnancies

most often, signs of impaired ovarian function rather than a fault of uterine growth. The role of imperfect paramesonephric duct fusion in the etiology of abortion is well known.

It has often been said that uterine myomas are associated with decreased fecundity but a really satisfactory explanation as to why intramural and subserous tumors interfere with reproduction has never been offered. It is easy to understand why a submucous tumor may do so. The endometrium over such a neoplasm is often so distorted that no self-respecting conceptus would ever consider implanting on it; or the tumor may, perhaps, act as an intrauterine device. Be that as it may, the diagnosis of lesser uterine anomalies, of endometrial synechiae and of uterine tumors, particularly submucous myomas, are essential considerations in infertility cases of obscure etiology. The value of hysteroroentgenography in the diagnosis of such problems (Fig. 2) is undisputed.

The technique of hysteroroentgenography is too well known to require discussion here. It may be well to emphasize, however, that overdistention of the uterus by the injected media or air bubbles in the uterine cavity may lead to erroneous diagnoses.

Hysterotomy may be required to confirm the roentgenographic diagnosis when there is a small submucous myoma that cannot be palpated manually.

The secretory activity of the endometrium is the mechanism which supplies the young conceptus with the nutritive substances it must have before and immediately after implantation. These substances are contained in the endometrial extracellular fluid and, presumably, the free fluid on the surface of the endometrium. Nutrients, vitamins and enzymes have been identified. The metabolism of some of these substances has been studied. That of the carbohydrates has been explored, particularly by EDWARD HUGHES. Alkaline phosphatase and glycogen in the endometrium and the secretion within the endometrial glands in the postovulatory phase apparently are responses to normal ovarian hormonal activity. HUGHES and his coworkers demonstrated aberrations in carbohydrate metabolism in the endometrium of patients with

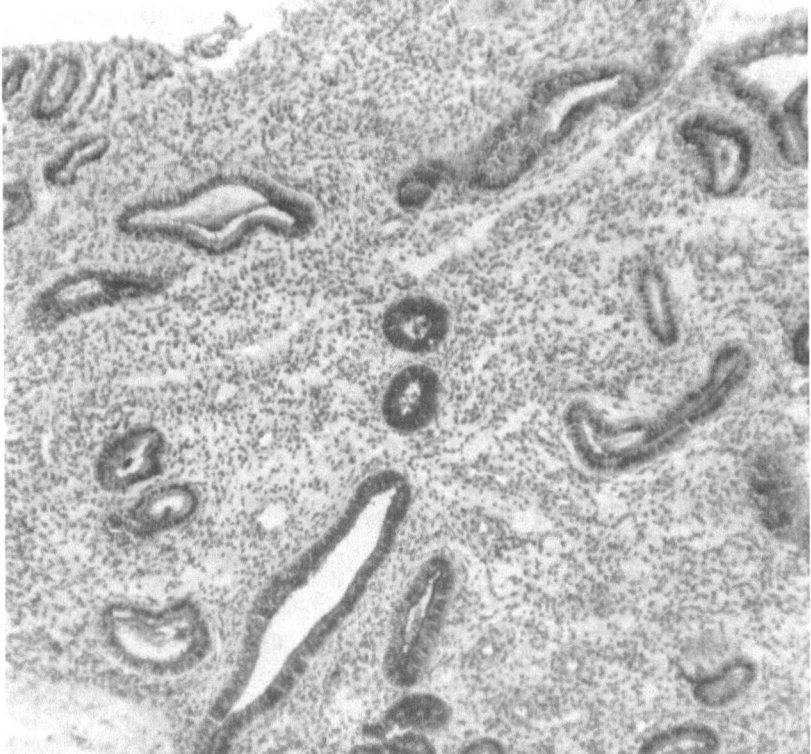

Fig. 3. The presence of alkaline phosphatase is indicated by dark granules in the epithelium and lumens of the endometrial glands (Gomori stain). From HUFFMAN, J.: Gynecology and Obstetrics. Philadelphia: W. B. Saunders Company 1962

histories of infertility and abortion. They found that the endometrium of women who were infertile contained an adequate amount of alkaline phosphatase but no glycogen. It is interesting to note that 84% of HUGHES' patients who were infertile showed a deficiency in endometrial glycogenesis although it did reveal secretory changes.

Studies of the histochemical reactions of the endometrium would therefore seem worthwhile in obscure problems of infertility. Endometrium for alkaline phosphatase and glycogen studies is obtained by biopsy on the 10. or 12. postovulatory day. The tissues are fixed in 95% alcohol. The Gomori technique is used to stain the sections to be examined for alkaline phosphatase (Fig. 3).

At the present time we have no way of determining the effect of the uterine secretions on the spermatozoa which migrate through the uterus on their way to the uterine tube. Presumably they are in a salutary environment. Nevertheless, relatively few male cells live to reach the uterine tube. The possibility that in some cases the secretions from the endometrial glands may have a deleterious effect on spermatozoa warrants consideration and would be a worthwhile subject for investigation.

The competency of the internal cervical os usually is not considered to be a necessary part of an infertility diagnostic study. It is not until the patient has suffered several late abortions or premature labors that incompetency of the internal os is suspected. The demonstration of a thin area in the upper portion of the anterior cervical wall by digital palpation over an intracervical dilator is highly suggestive. I also wish to mention the value of hysterography in making the diagnosis of an incompetent internal os (Fig. 4).

We have made relatively little progress in the diagnosis of cervical factors in infertility since J. MARION SIMS (1866) first described the examination of postcoital cervical secretion. The identification of appreciable numbers of motile spermatozoa in cervical mucus for a number of hours after coitus is proof not only that there is no cervical barrier to sperm migration but that the sperm themselves are viable and, presumably, fertile. The value of the Sims-Huhner test as an index of the husband's fecundity, ideally performed after 4 days of continence, is not sufficiently appreciated. Furthermore, the admonition that one negative test may be misleading is not always kept in mind.

In vitro study of the penetration of the cervical secretions by the spermatozoa is of value when repeated Sims-Huhner tests are unsatisfactory. The simple procedure consists of placing a drop of the husband's seminal fluid inside a ring of cervical mucus. Microscopic examination of the preparation will give some idea of the interaction between the sperm and the cervical secretion. Failure of penetration by the spermatozoa presumably may be caused by hostile factors in the cervical mucus or the spermatozoa may be weak. The test does not differentiate between the two. Control preparations can be made using the husband's sperm and the cervical secretion from a women who is known to be fertile or by using the wife's secretion and seminal fluid from a fertile man. Such tests are not conclusive; they are helpful in those unusual instances where a cervical factor is thought to be responsible for the patient's infertility.

The presence of glairy, crystalline cervical mucus demonstrating *Spinnbarkeit* during the ovulatory phase of the cycle (Fig. 5) is an obvious indicator of cervical normalcy. The formation of fern-like patterns in the dried mucus at the time of ovulation, as demonstrated by LA PAZ, is a further indicator that the cervical secretions are normal. Such secretions presumably favor sperm migration. On the other hand, the cervical canal, when filled with a thick, viscid secretion at midcycle, may be a barrier instead of a passageway for the spermatozoa. Obviously, study of the cervical mucus and evaluation of the cervical secretions are important parts of the examination of the infertile women.

The possibility that clear, crystalline cervical mucus could, of itself, be hostile to spermatozoa would seem inconceivable yet there are patients who seem to exhibit

526

such a state. Although its chemical composition is not precisely known, cervical mucus exhibits several specific characteristics. Those characteristics which are best understood have to do with its physical rheological properties. But these are not specific. *Spinnbarkeit* varies from patient to patient and from cycle to cycle. Fern

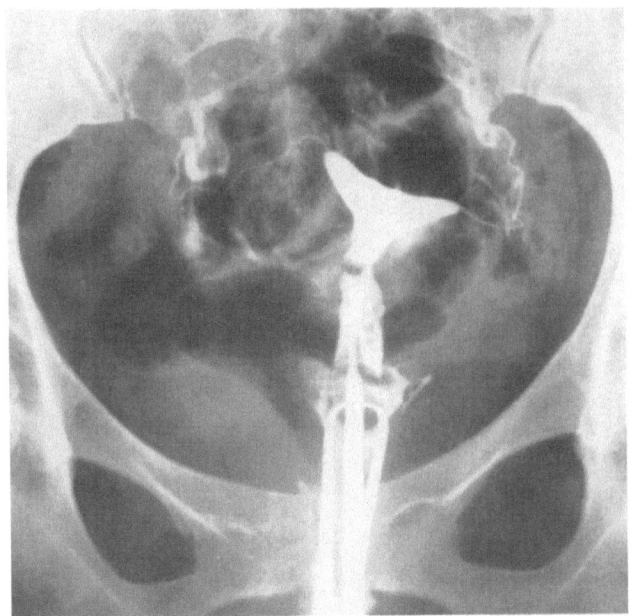

Fig. 4. Incompetent internal cervical os. Patient had had four late abortions. The isthmic canal measures more than 1 cm in width. An incompetent os was demonstrated surgically. Following cervicoplasty she had an uneventful term pregnancy

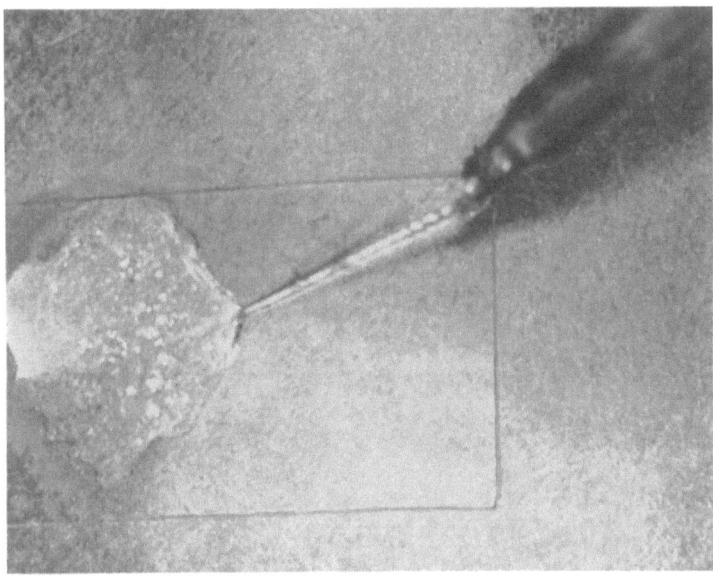

Fig. 5. *Spinnbarkeit* is demonstrated by lifting a thread of cervical secretion from a glass slide with a pipet

formation depends on electrolyte concentration and is not necessarily an indicator of specific organic events. It occurs, however, under the influence of estrogen and often does not occur in mucus from infected glands. We have yet to develop the sophisticated techniques which are needed to determine the chemical, enzymatic and immuno-

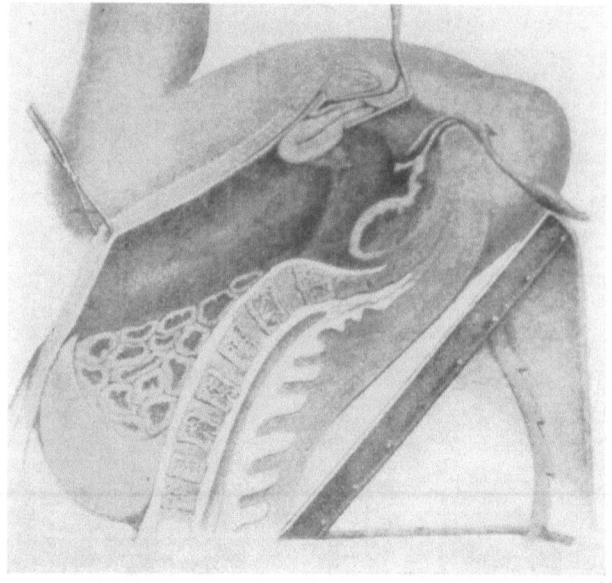

A

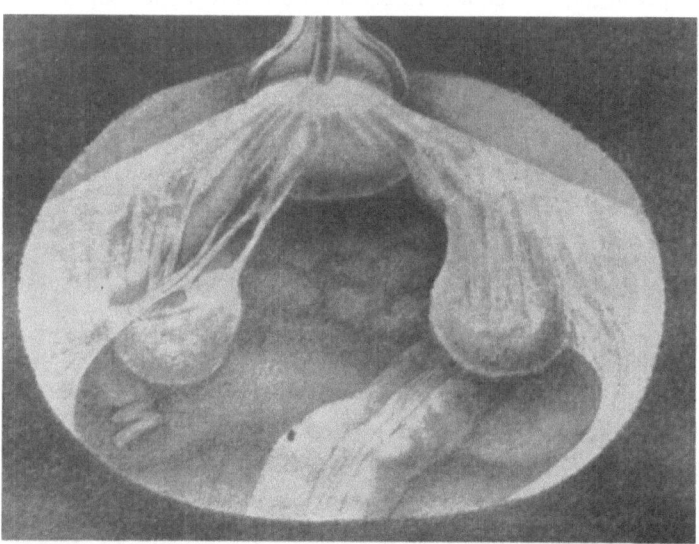

B

Fig. 6. A—B. Colpotomy for visualization of the pelvic viscera was first described by von Ott (1903). A Illustration from von Ott's original paper showing wide colpotomy incision, use of long vaginal retractors and patient's pelvis markedly elevated. B An illustration from von Ott's paper demonstrating the ease with which the pelvis could be visualized; there are adhesions about the uterine tubes and ovaries

logical reactions of the cervical mucus. We will not be able to deal competently with cervical factors in infertility until the exact composition of normal and pathological cervical mucus is known as well as the process for their biosynthesis.

Many things may alter normal cervical secretions and interfere with sperm migration. Most often the absence of crystalline midcycle secretion indicates defective hormonal stimulation. The role of chronic endocervicitis in the interference of sperm migration merits emphasis. Chronic infections, whether they are secondary to partial obstruction and poor drainage or are residues of specific disease, may cause a persistent mucopurulent discharge which blocks the cervical canal. The inflammatory reactions interfere with the normal alterations in the cervical secretion. Conization or other surgery on the cervix and excessive electrical and chemical cauterization may destroy the cervical mucosa with the loss of necessary cervical secretion.

I find it difficult to accept the thesis that cervical polyps, a small cervical os or a nabothian follicle cyst will block a cervical canal to the point where the spermatozoa cannot find a passageway. Admittedly, the long, narrow, adolescent type of cervix with a pin-point os which is characteristic of uterine hypoplasia may be inimical to sperm transport but such a structure, in most cases, is the result of ovarian hypofunction rather than failure of cervical development.

There are, in addition, occasional instances when the diagnosis of uterotubal factors which adversely affect reproduction may not be evident by insufflation or hysterosalpingography. In these diagnostic problems culdoscopy, devised by DECKER, and colpotomy are of value. Culdoscopy has the advantage of simplicity, of returning the patient to her normal activities within a short time and of safety. Use of fiber optic sources has improved the clarity and extent of visualization and tubal and ovarian disease can be diagnosed with considerable accuracy.

Colpotomy, first described by VON OTT (1903), has the disadvantage of being a surgical procedure which requires several days' hospitalization. It is, however, associated with a minimal degree of surgical risk and gives the operator not only excellent visualization of the internal genitalia (Fig. 6) but also the opportunity to perform necessary corrective procedures.

There are cases in which every diagnostic procedure has been performed without uncovering a reason for the patient's infertility. Exploratory laparotomy merits consideration in carefully selected cases of this type because unsuspected uterine, tubal or ovarian pathology will be uncovered in an appreciable number of them.

Conclusion

The physician, when he considers the role of uterotubal factors in infertility and sterility, needs to know whether the patient's cervical canal affords a friendly environment for the passage of spermatozoa, whether the region of the internal os is competent to retain a conceptus within the uterine cavity, whether the endometrium offers a favorable environment for its growth and whether the uterine tubes not only are unobstructed avenues for the transport of the zygote but also have the necessary peristalic movements to propel the ovum on its way. He has available a number of roentgenographic and other techniques to help him assess the patient's reproductive potential. This has been a brief and necessarily panoramic review of those techniques. The procedures mentioned included: Sims-Huhner postcoital test; in vitro study of cervical-seminal hostility; study of the rheological and physical characteristics of the cervical secretions; roentgenographic study of cervical competency; hysterography;

histochemical study of endometrium; endometrial culture; uterotubal insufflation; uterotubal perfusion; hysterosalpingography; culdoscopy; colpotomy and laparatomy.

References

Bang, J.: Acta obstet. gynec. scand. **29,** 383 (1950).
Béclère, C., et G. Fayolle: L'Hystérosalpingographie. Paris: Masson et Cie 1961.
Buxton, C. L., and L. Mastroianni: Fertil. and Steril. **14,** 284 (1963).
Carey, W. H.: Amer. J. Obstet. Dis. Wom. **69,** 462 (1914).
Cohen, M. R., I. F. Stein, and B. M. Kaye: Fertil. and Steril. **3,** 201 (1952).
Decker, A.: Culdoscopy. Philadelphia: F. A. Davis: 1967.
—, and T. Cherry: Amer. J. Surg. **64,** 40 (1944).
de Paz, A. C., Jr.: Fertil. and Steril. **4,** 137 (1953).
Goldbert, B., and H. W. Jones: Proc. Soc. exp. Biol. (N.Y.) **83,** 45 (1953).
Heuser, C.: Lancet **1925 II,** 1111.
Hughes, E. C.: Amer. J. Obstet. Gynec. **49,** 10 (1945).
Jeffcoate, T. N. A., and J. K. Wetson: N. Y. St. J. Med. **56,** 680 (1956).
Johnstone, J. W.: J. Obstet. Gynec. Brit. Emp. **65,** 208 (1958).
Lash, A. F., and S. R. Lash: Amer. J. Obstet. Gynec. **59,** 68 (1950).
Ludlow, I.: Cleveland med. J. **8,** 398 (1909).
Palmer, R., et M. Lacomme: Gynéc. et Obstét. **47,** 905 (1948).
Platt, H. A.: Ann. N.Y. Acad. Sci. **130,** 925 (1966).
Pommerenke, W. T.: Amer. J. Obstet. Gynec. **52,** 1032 (1946).
Pocher, P., et J. Varangot: Bull. Fed. Gynéc. Obstrt. franç. **7,** 44 (1955).
Pullman, I., and J. S. Laughlin: Gonadal dose produced by the medical use of X-rays. National Acad. Sci., Nat. Research Council, Washington 1957.
Rindfleisch, W.: Klin. Wschr. **47,** 780 (1910).
Röntgen, W. C.: S.-B. physik. med. Ges. Wurzburg **137,** 132 (1895).
Rubin, I. C.: Zbl. Gynäk. **38,** 658 (1914).
— Amer. J. Obstet. Gynec. **14,** 557 (1927).
Rubovits, F. G., N. R. Cooperman, and A. F. Lash: Amer. J. Obstet. Gynec. **66,** 269 (1953).
Siegler, A. M.: Fertil. and Steril. **6,** 432 (1955).
— Hysterosalpingography. New York: Haeber Medical Division, Harper and Row, Publishers 1967.
Stallworthy, J.: Fertil. and Steril. **14,** 284 (1963).
Stein, I. F.: Surg. Gynec. Obstet. **42,** 83 (1926).
—, and R. A. Arens: Amer. J. Obstet. Gynec. **18,** 130 (1929).
Tompkins, P. T.: Amer. J. Obstet. Gynec. **83,** 1599 (1962).
von Ott, D.: Mschr. Geburtsh. Gynäk. **18,** 645 (1903).

Utero-tubal Insufflation and Perfusion

R. Fikentscher

The diagnostic grasp of the tubal factor as the cause of female sterility presents many problems today. We have to keep in mind that the present available methods of examination may discover the impassibility of the tubes. But in no way can they show us other disorders of the physiological functions of the tubes which may be important in the occurrance of pregnancy. In other words we can discover very well the different forms of mechanical obstructions in the medium of transportation which the tubes represent. We cannot say with certainty anything about the finer functions of the tubes; for example, whether they are capable enough to transport and nourish the eggs. (Their importance was presented in the report of Dr. Mulligan.)

Of course the discovery, the prognostic judgement and the possible elimination of the mechanical obstructions in the tubes play a dominant role in the treatment of sterility. In the following we will show the diagnostic procedure of the Second Frauenklinik of the University of Munich and how we are endeavouring to expand the therapeutic possibilities with hydropertubation.

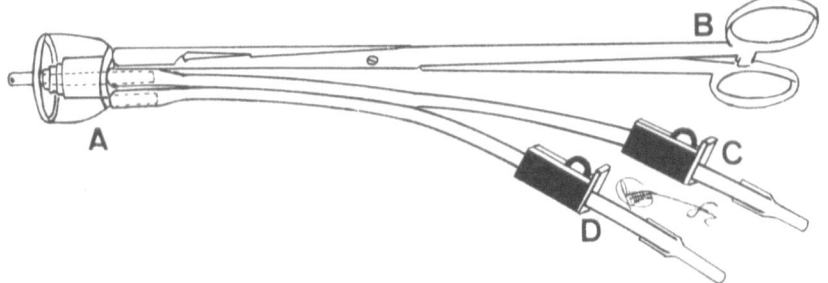

Fig. 1 A—D. Cervix Adapter according to FIKENTSCHER and SEMM for insufflation of carbon-dioxide gas, hysterosalpingography or hydropertubation (flexible disposable instrument made of transparent plastic). A Cervix Adapter bell, B forceps to direct the Cervix Adapter into the vagina, C insufflation tube with "roll-on" clamp, D Vacuum tube with "roll-on" clamp

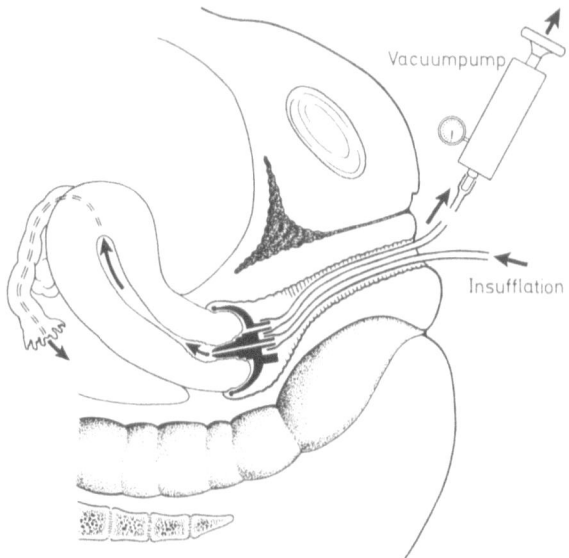

Fig. 2. Cervix Adapter according to FIKENTSCHER and SEMM in situ. The flexible instrument seals the cervical canal by suction and is used for carbon-dioxide gas pertubation, hysterosalpingography and hydropertubation

For the patency test of the tubes *the utero-tubal insufflation* is of primary importance in our clinic:

After sealing the cervical canal, carbon dioxide gas is blown through the uterus and the tubes. The pressure and the quantity of the carbon dioxide gas are precisely controlled by an apparatus (Fig. 1).

Our cervix-adapter serves as the sealing instrument. Together with its flexible tubes it forms a handy system and seals the cervical canal through suction (Fig. 2).

The low pressure is produced by a little vacuum pump and controlled with a mano-meter. The cervix-adapter is a disposable instrument.

The suction on the portio causes neither tissue damage nor pain. The examination can be performed without narcosis. The flexible tubes present no change in the topo-graphical position of the uterus and the adnexes.

The necessary pressure for persufflation of the tubes is produced by our universal pertubation apparatus (Fig. 3). The pressure increase is fractionated, starting with

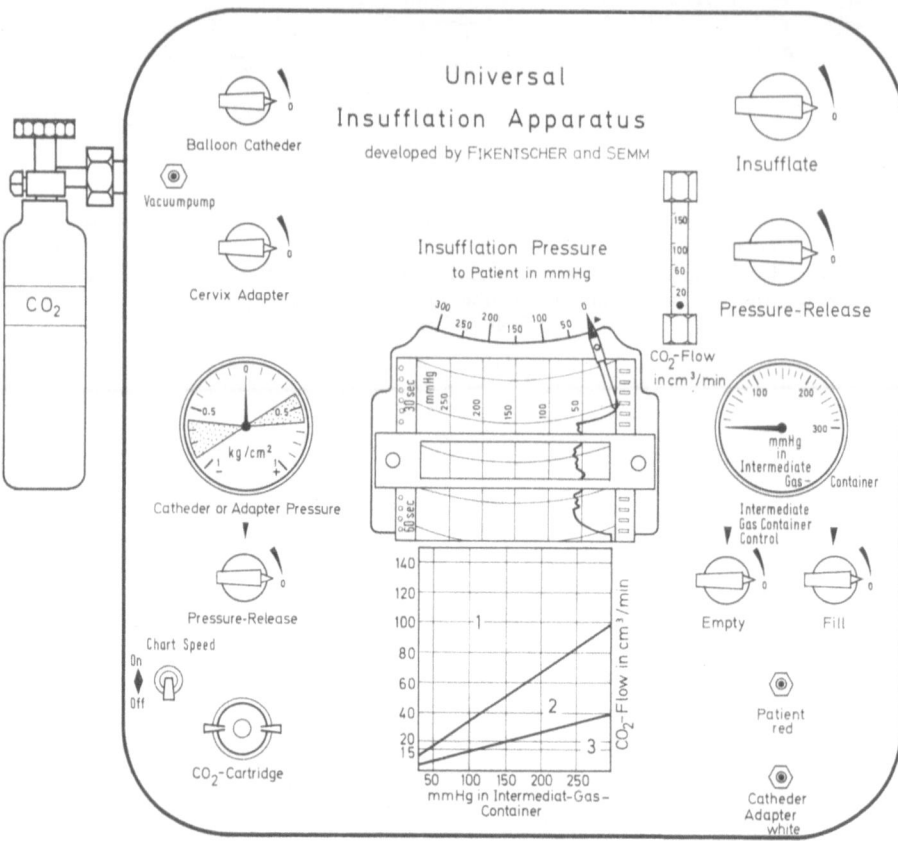

Fig. 3. Universal Pertubation Apparatus according to FIKENTSCHER and SEMM with graphic registration of the pressure values during the carbon dioxide gas insufflation; atraumatic sealing of the cervical canal by double-balloon-catheter or Cervix Adapter

50 mm of mercury. The suspension height of the ball in the flow meter (Fig. 4) indi-cates how many ccm of carbon dioxide gas flow through the tubes into the abdomen. Corresponding to the suspension height of the ball we are able to infer from our diagram the following degrees of patency:

1. normal patency,
2. difficult patency,
3. and stenosed patency.

The comparison of the obtained oscillogram with its characteristic curve traces makes a broad diagnostic possible (Fig. 5).

Consequently, there are specific curve pictures which are very typical of the different morphological and functional changes of the tubes. The characteristic oscillogram:

by normal bilateral tubal patency,

by unilateral tubal patency,

by tubal or uteral spasm,

by tubal stenosis,

by unilateral or bilateral hydrosalpinx,

by intramural occlusion.

The eventual occurrence of pain during the insufflation together with such oscillograms are important differential diagnostic hints: If the insufflation of carbon dioxide gas up to 300 mm of mercury is possible without any special reference of pain on the part of the patient, it is highly probable that the occlusion is intramural. The gas in the uterus is only felt as dull pressure. However, if the patient complains of pain at a pressure of 100 to 150 mm of mercury, the occlusion is without a doubt

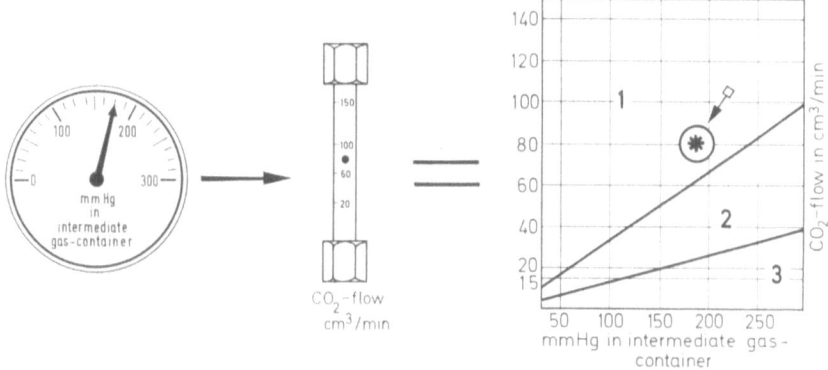

Fig. 4. Determination of the degree of tubal patency by two values: insufflation pressure (in this case the manometer shows 180 mm of mercury) and gas flow (in this case 80 ml/min). The diagram shows the first degree of tubal patency for both values

peripheral. Peritoneal pain develops from tubal inflation. We observe these peritoneal pains from hydrosalpinx, from peripheral occlusions and from peritubal adhesions. These different tubal changes show different diagrams.

The diagrammatic indications and the degree of persufflation in connection with the pain diagnostic are very valuable.

The presented technique of a utero-tubal insufflation represents the smallest degree of a surgical procedure necessary to clarify the tubal factor. This technique makes it possible for us to acquire essential information about the tubal situation and, therefore, in our clinic it is the first diagnostic stage in the clarification of the tubal factor.

Surely the utero-tubal insufflation is not able to give definite information relative to some questions, for instance concerning the relationships of the tubal ostia to the ovary and the eventually existing obstructions there. In spite of these obstructions, sometimes almost normal diagrams are obtained.

As a further diagnosis of utero-tubal patency *the hysterosalpingography* is at our disposal. We are again using our flexible cervix-adapter which even for this purpose does not change the topographical situation. In addition it also makes possible a

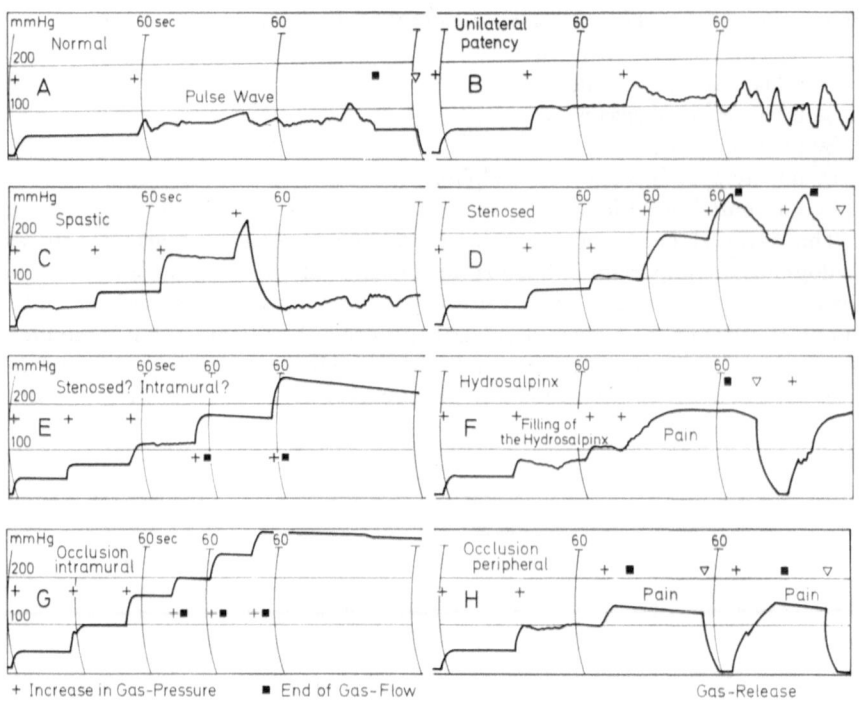

+ Increase in Gas-Pressure   ■ End of Gas-Flow   Gas-Release

Fig. 5 A—H. Curve-traces obtained by pertubation of the tubes with the Universal In-sufflation Apparatus by FIKENTSCHER and SEMM. A Normal bilateral patency of the tubes. After increase in pressure step by step for 1 min from 50 mm Hg to 75—100 mm Hgthe graph shows shallow oscillations modulated by oscillations of a higher frequency equal to the pulse frequency. Flow is 120 ml per min at 300 mm Hg in the intercontainer. B Unilateral patency of the tubes. The gas passage is set at 100 mm Hg. After a gradual increase of the pressure to 110 mm Hg the graph shows high amplitudes, which are also modulated by pulse-waves. Flow is 100 ml per min at 300 mm Hg in the intercontainer. C Spasm of the tubes or the uterus. With spastic patients the pressure can be painlessly increased to 200 to 250 mm Hg step by step in intervals of 1 min each. A sudden decrease of the pressure graph and flow, as in A, is typical. D, E Peripheral or intramural stenosis. During gradual increase of the pressure the graph already shows a slight gas flow at 100 mm Hg. After the gas is stopped, the flow graph slopes down at an angle of about 45 degrees. Flow is less than 40 ml per min at 300 mm Hg in the intercontainer. F Unilateral or bilateral hydrosalpinx. After a graduated increase of pressure the graph at first is normal. The trace, however, soon flattens out. In most cases the insufflation has to be stopped at 150 mm Hg because the pain becomes unbearable. If insufflation is repeated, a sudden increase of pressure causes pain as the tubes are still filled with gas. G Intramural occlusion of the tubes. After each increase of pressure the graph shows a straight trace in the same pressure range. The slight pressure decrease after the gas flow is stopped is caused by the gas resorption by the endometrium. H Peripheral occlusion of the tubes. After a graduated increase of the pressure to about 100 mm Hg a further increase of pressure to 150 mm Hg or at most 200 mm Hg causes unbearable pain. This can be repeatedly reproduced by releasing the gas and then increasing the pressure to 150 or 200 mm Hg. A and F Peritubal intergrowths. If the pain already starts during procedure A after 1.5 to 2 min or earlier and is unilateral or bilateral without a decrease in the flowing gas volume (as in F), the diagnosis is peritubal intergrowths. This phenomenon will be observed in most cases after an insufflated gas volume of 150 cc. In these cases the shoulder pain will be observed to be delayed or will not occur at all

clear observation of the cervical canal and the configuration of the entire uterus cavity in the contrast picture. The course of the tubes and their patency are diagnosed either immediately with the X-ray screen or in the X-ray picture (through the first or later pictures after 30 to 60 min).

The type of spreading of the contrast substance in the lesser or true pelvis gives valuable hints. Sharp straight lined shadows of the contrast substance indicate perisalpingitic adhesions (Fig. 6).

Even the HSG cannot give definite information about the anatomic-functional connections of the tubes, especially their ampulla ends to the ovaries and the other neighboring organs. Therefore, and because of possible actinogene injuries, we normally use it only in cases for the necessary clarification of the cervix and uterus cavity situation in the form of a hysterography.

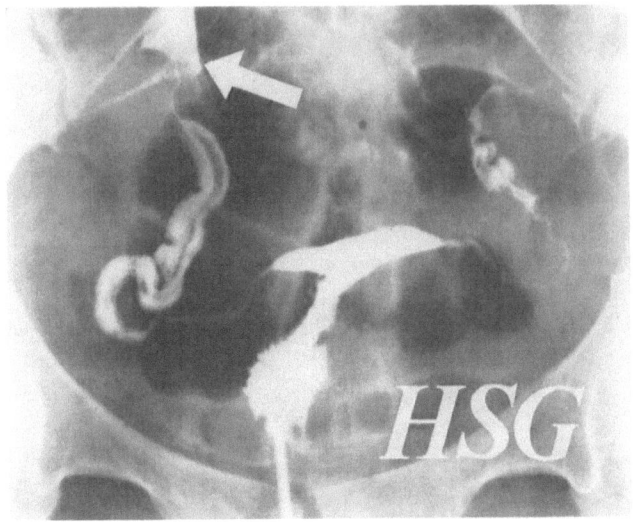

Fig. 6. Hysterosalpingography of 32 year old woman. The hysterosalpingogram gives a precise picture of the lumina of cervix, uterus and tubes. The straightlined shadows (mark) indicate perisalpingitic adhesions. An exact diagnosis of these adhesions, however, can not be made by hysterosalpingography

In view of the prognosis and the assessment of the chances of success of surgical treatment of a tubal factor, we regard *the gynecological pelviscopy* as the best diagnostic method.

In association with our carbon dioxide persufflation or a chromopertubation we are in the position to answer the above mentioned questions.

The gynecological pelviscopy, still widely regarded as very severe, relatively dangerous and technically difficult, has become a routine method today due to the essential improvement of the instruments.

The technique developed by SEMM in my clinic makes use of the following:

1. The navel pit is the portal of entry for the carbon dioxide gas and for the pelviscope (Fig. 7).

2. Three technical improvements:

a) The cold light, in spite of its high illumination, does not endanger the body cavity.

b) The optic with its extremely small systems makes it possible to construct very thin pelviscopes.

c) Through the automatisation of the gas filling process, a false inflow of the gas is immediately indicated on the apparatus.

3. A newly developed inflexible perforated vacuum intrauterine sound by SEMM (Fig. 8) is sucked by means of low pressure on to the portio vaginalis. The instrument

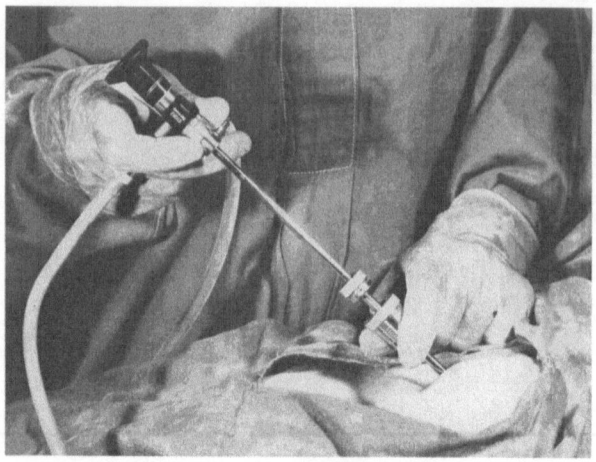

Fig. 7. Introduction of a 4 mm Hopkins-endoscope through the navel pit for "Gynecological Pelviscopy". The abdominal cavity is filled with carbon-dioxide gas, using the CO_2-Pneu-Automatic according to SEMM

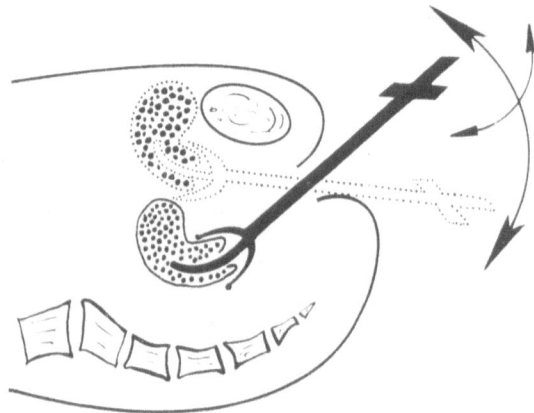

Fig. 8. Vacuum intrauterine sound developed by SEMM, permitting the three-dimensional movement of the uterus during the "Gynecological Pelviscopy". Carbon-dioxide gas or indigocarmine solution can be brought into the uterine cavity by the multiperforated intrauterine sound

permits the movement of the uterus in different directions during endoscopic observation and simultaneously insufflates gas or blue colored solution as a test of tubal patency. The mobility of the uterus by means of the sound, for example by elevating it and the additional chromopertubation (Fig. 9), permit an exhaustive observation with the pelviscope.

The perfusion of liquids through Müller's ducts has been used for many years as the only or additional diagnostic method. Hydropertubation (perfusion) as a remedy has become increasingly important in latter times. We obtain an essential improvement through *"repeated long acting-hydropertubation"*. Considering that the instilled solutions with the generally used techniques of hydropertubation remain only a short time in the genital tract, we developed a special method. In principle the instilled

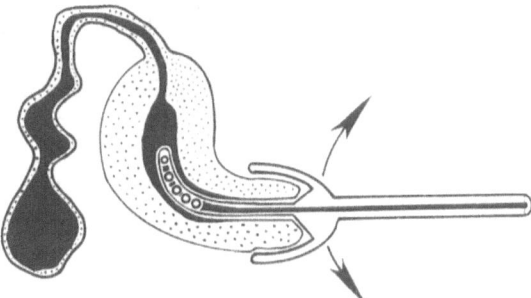

Fig. 9. Chromopertubation: The uterine cavity and the sactosalpinx are filled with blue solution at a pressure of 150 mm mercury. The endoscopic observation shows a thick blue tube. The "Gynecological Pelviscopy" in connection with the Chromopertubation allow a perfect diagnostic evaluation of the Fallopian tubes

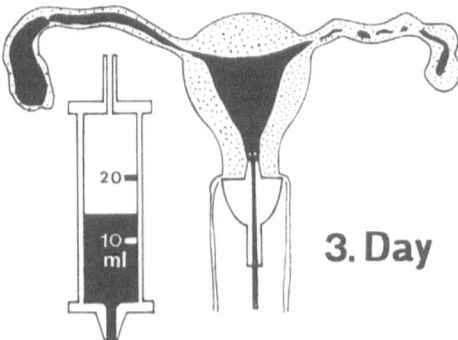

Fig. 10. Repeated Long-acting Hydropertubation: situation on the third day: 7 ml are instilled. The liquid has reached the ampullary end of the right tube, the left tube shows only a slightly filled lumen

solution *remains* for several hours (on the average 6 to 8 h) in those places where the therapeutic effects are desired (Fig. 10) and a *repetition* of such instillations is performed 6 or 8 days in the first half of the cycle.

Again we use our flexible disposable cervix-adapter which by means of low pressure is sucked onto the portio vaginalis. The instillation of the solution succeeds under a controlled pressure of 100 to 200 mm of mercury. The reflux of the solution is prevented as long as the adapter is not removed (Fig. 11).

The following instillation solution consisting of a mixture of 0.4 g of streptomycin-sulfate, 0.01 g of hydrocortison-acetate and 0.04 g of procaine-hydrochloride with the addition of 10 ml of distilled water has been approved by us.

In addition 25 C.Hb.E. α-chymotrypsin are dissolved in 5 ml of distilled water. Consequently this mixture has a combined antibacterial, antiphlogistic and fibrinolytic effect.

Especially, we want to mention that a repeated long acting-hydropertubation with our technique is well tolerated:

1. The procedure causes no special pains, as the instilled solution contains procaine and the vacuum fixating the adapter is decreased after the instillation.

2. We never observed a new or recurrent adnexitis.

3. Furthermore, by often repeated long acting-hydropertubation we found no evidence of local or general injury.

We perform our repeated long acting-hydropertubation as a preoperative as well as a postoperative measure, sometimes even as a single therapy without any surgical procedure. In one case we start the instillation immediately after menstruation, and in the other case the first or second day after the tubal operation.

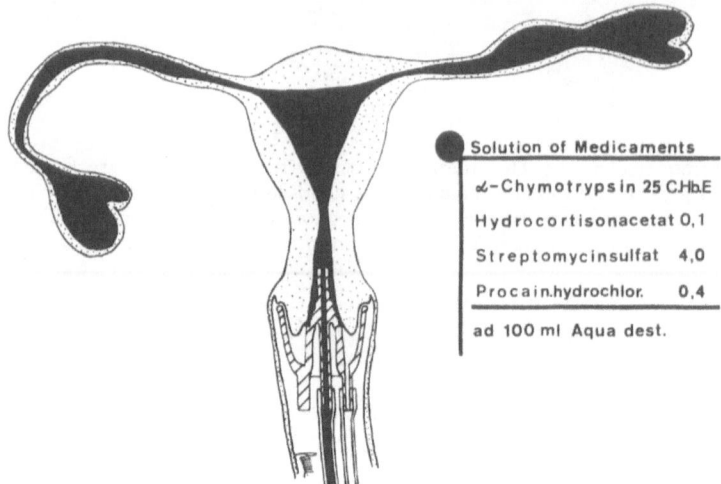

Fig. 11. Principle of the Long-acting Hydropertubation: Liquid is instilled into the tubes and the uterine cavity using the Cervix Adapter. The Cervix Adapter prevents the reflux of the solution for 6 to 8 h. During this procedure the vacuum for fixing the Cervix Adapter to the portio vaginalis is being lowered to —0.1 kg/cm²

The success of hydropertubation series on the obstructed tubes can be proved by the daily increasing quantity of the instillation. Usually the break through of the therapy solution into the free abdominal cavity occurs on the 5th or 6th day.

By the introduction of repeated long acting-hydropertubation the rate of postoperative tubes remaining open has increased considerably. In our operative material by the test of tubal patency with carbon dioxide gas after the third to fifth postoperative cycle the rate of re-occluded tubes decreased from 25% to nearly 10%. After we began to treat every tubal sterility operation with repeated long acting-hydropertubation the frequency of open tubes increased from 76% to 90%.

Our reported diagnostic method of utero-tubal insufflation and the repeated long acting hydropertubation is further illustrated in our films "The tubal diagnostic" and "The hydropertubation therapy".

References

FIKENTSCHER, R.: Geburtsh. u. Frauenheilk. **26**, 686 (1966).
— Z. Geburtsh. Gynäk. Suppl. **168**, 168 (1968).
—, u. K. SEMM: Geburtsh. u. Frauenheilk. **15**, 313 (1955).

— — Présentation d'un Appareil Universel pour I.U.T. et H.S.G. In: Société nationale pour l'étude de la Stérilité et de la Fécondité. La Fonction tubaire et ses Troubles, p. 65. Paris: Masson et Cie. 1956.

— — Arch. Gynäk. **188**, 184 (1956).

— — Gynéc. prat. **9**, 413 (1958).

— — Geburtsh. u. Frauenheilk. **18**, 161 (1958).

— — Beitrag zur Deutung der bei der utero-tubaren Persufflation erhaltenen Oscillationen. Proceedings of the IV. World Congress on Fertility and Sterility Vol. I., p. 949. Neapel 1958.

— — Geburtsh. u. Frauenheilk. **19**, 868 (1959).

— — Z. Geburtsh. Gynäk. **155**, 215 (1960).

MOHR, A. R., e J. GOMES DA SILVEIRA: Rev. Assoc. méd. Rio Gr. Sul **4**, 111 (1960).

SEMM, K.: Prüfung der Tubendurchgängigkeit. In: FRIEDBERG, V. F., K. G. OBER, K. THOMSEN und J. ZANDER, Gynäkologie und Geburtshilfe, Vol. 1, p. 272. Stuttgart: Thieme 1968.

— Geburtsh. u. Frauenheilk. **27**, 1029 (1967).

— Diagnostic methods. In: BEHRMAN, S. J., and R. KISTNER, Progress in infertility, chapt. X/39. Boston/Mass.: Little Brown & Comp. 1968.

Restorative Surgery of the Tubes

(a study of 600 personal cases)

RAOUL PALMER

Organic obstruction of the tubes is still in France the most frequent factor of persistent sterility (around 40%). *Pelvic adhesions* are also an important factor, isolated in 5 to 10%, associated with organic obstruction in 25% at least.

Statistical Evaluation of Results

My *personal global statistic* from 1942 to 1961, published in Vienna in 1964, included 489 tuboplasties, 306 with patency (62%), 105 with uterine pregnancy (21%) and 30 with extra-uterine pregnancy (6%).

Results by category of operation are much more difficult to establish, because quite often a different operation has been done on the right and the left side, and, if a uterine pregnancy occurs, it is difficult to assess which operation was successful. Therefore, we have selected, from our personal statistics until 1965, 600 unequivocal cases, where the same operation has been done on both sides (or on one side, the other tube being removed).

Pre-Operative Explorations

A recent hysterosalpingography with hydrosolubles is compulsory to visualize perfectly a) *the interstitial part of the tube* (especially in cases of proximal occlusion); b) *the folds of the ampulla* (if they are very irregular, the danger of tubal pregnancy is great).

A search for signs of latent tuberculosis is very important (we find in France 16% proved and 20% probable tuberculosis, and the results among 110 such cases operated by me, are: 2 tubal and *no* uterine pregnancy).

Laparoscopy is compulsory in cases of proximal occlusion (as more than 60% are associated with distal pathology); it is also very useful in distal occlusion, as it is the only way (besides laparotomy) to know the state of fimbria and ovary and the extension and density of adhesions. In most cases, we perform the laparotomy *just before* the operation.

Absolute contra-indications to tuboplasty were:

1. the known tuberculous origin of the obstruction; 2. other important and persistant factors in man or women; 3. tubes with narrow ampulla or multiple strictions at salpingography; 4. very dense adhesions at laparoscopy; 5. age above 37.

Temporary contra-indications were:

1. Subacute inflammation; 2. tubal pregnancy: in such cases we postpone tuboplasty for some months.

Tuboplasty must be as atraumatic as possible; the mucosa should never be caught with a forceps; any distension or traction should be avoided; atraumatic needles with 0000 nylon, or other non-reactive material, should be used. The instruments we use are those designed for ophthalmologic surgery. Gentleness and minutia are compulsory.

Operation is done just after menstruation, through a low Pfannenstiel incision; the uterus is anchored with two catguts placed in cross on the top.

Salpingolysis

Salpingolysis (the operative liberation of adhesions) is the first, and very important step. It should always be done under *total visual control* (changing side when necessary), and by section or resection with Knife or Scissors and never with the fingers.

It must be carried out methodically:

1. *The omentum* should first be separated completely from abdominal wall, bladder, uterus, tube and ovary;

2. *The intestines* should then be dissected cautiously, with immediate repair, if any injury;

3. *The adnexa* should be separated from the uterus and ligamentum latum progressively, with maximal caution at the inferior pole, where the end of the tube is often imbedded in dense adhesions.

Then, the whole adnexa can be brought upwards and the careful separation of the tube from the ovary is performed. Then the ovary is thoroughly "cleaned" from adhesive remnants. Adhesions between tubal loops are mostly respected, except when there is compression by a true fibrous band (v.i.).

Salpingolysis may sometimes be the whole operation.

In 26 cases of *bilateral* operative Salpingolysis for sterility of more than 3 years duration, we had 14 uterine pregnancies (56%) — most of them in the year.

Per-operative Exploration

Thorough per-operative exploration of the tubes includes:

1. *Inspection* of the distal end, to see what remains of the infundibulum; 2. *palpation*, to locate the indurated or thickened areas; 3. exploration of the infundibulum and ampulla with a No. 10 Nelaton catheter.

True study of patency should only be performed if doubt persists between *organic* or *spasmodic* stenosis or occlusion of the proximal portion of the tube. In such cases, we perform hydrotubation with Shirodkar's technique, but using blue dye and manometric control. If any doubt about spasm persists, I amp. hydergin is injected intra-venously.

A *tubal biopsy* should be done every time the operation is not confined to blunt separation of agglutinated fimbria, either by sending the resected parts, or taking a strip on the margin of section. The tubal biopsy is very important for the management of postoperative treatment, as it may show unsuspected tuberculosis, inflammatory active sclerosis, endometriosis, etc. *The importance of inflammatory sclerosis* must be emphazised: in a series of 108 ampullar salpin gostomies (in a study presented at Stockholm with JEAN DE BRUX in 1966) this pathology was present in 28 cases, with 22 re-occlusions, 1 E.U.P. (extra-uterine pregnancy) and only 1 U.P. (uterine pregnancy). On the contrary, 45 cases with simple sclerosis, gave only 14 re-occlusions, 9 U.P. and 6 E.U.P.

Codonolysis

Codonolysis (or fimbriolysis) consists in the blunt separation of agglutinated fimbriae, leading to the reshapening of the original ostium. It is the operation which gives the best results, everytime it is possible.

Sometimes, we find only *phimosis* of the infundibulum, and one can introduce into it a very fine Leriche forceps, and open it in various diameters, to de-agglutinate the fimbrial folds.

On other occasions, the peritoneal cover is continuous, but, after distension of the ampulla with hydrotubation, a slight depression, or a blue spot marks the site of the preexisting ostium. In such cases, Shirodkar's technique consists of crucial incision of the peritoneum alone (1 cm for each branch) and then the *codonolysis* as above described. Four stitches may help persistent extroversion of the fimbriae.

Our results with true codonolysis are, among 56 cases, 41 with patency (75%), 16 U.P. (29%) and 5 E.U.P. (9%).

Salpingostomy

Salpingostomy is the creation of a new opening in the tube, with or without resection of a part of it. It may be terminal, ampullar or isthmic.

Some facts should be remembered:

1. Persistence of a well patent ostium is a sine qua non condition of success.

2. There should also be some substitute to the fimbriae, that is some exterior mucous surface, with ciliated cells, to help the capture of the ovum.

3. It should preferably be in a position facilitating this capture.

4. The preserved portion of the ampulla should be sane.

But one should, cut away only the very dilated parts (more than the thumb), or the very thickened or sclerotic ones.

Terminal salpingostomy is done when the distal part of the tube is neither thickened nor too much distended. In most cases, we use a variant of Bonney's cuff technique: after vertical incision of the tubal end we put Bonney's clamp, and a cuff is easily obtained, and fixed with 5 or 6 well anchored stitches of nylon 0000 (Fig. 1).

When the cuff is impossible, we use Pollosson's technique, longitudinal dorsal incision, 25 to 30 mm long, and eversion of the mucosa by 8 to 12 stitches; the most distal stitch fixes the racket-shaped new ostium to the surface of the ovary (Fig. 2).

541

Among 123 cases of terminal salpingostomy of our 51 to 65 private patient series, we find 94 patencies (77%), 34 U.P. (27%) and 16 U.E.P. (13%). The results are about the same with the two varients.

Ampullar salpingostomy, though avoided when possible, is frequent in our series (148 cases).

Here too, we perform, when possible, a variant of *Bonney's cuff operation*, which we described in London in 1959: clamping of the ampulla as distally as possible; section and hemostasis of the meso salpinx; circular section of the peritoneum 2 cm from the clamp; section of the tube just besides the clamp; removal of the peritoneal cylinder; placing of Bonney's or Caplier's tubal clamp; making the cuff, and fixing it with

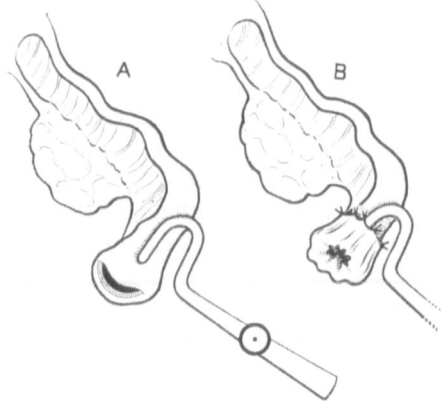

Fig. 1. Terminal salpingostomy by Bonney's cuff technique

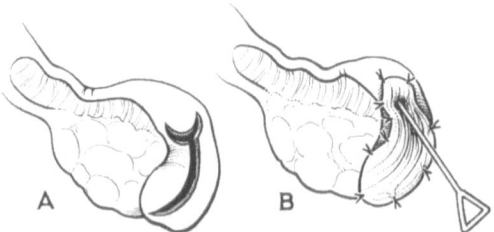

Fig. 2. Terminal salpingostomy ny Pollosson's racket technique

5 to 6 stitches of nylon 0000. Reconstruction of the tubo-ovarian ligament. The reason to remove the peritoneal cylinder is that it is the peritoneum which prevents the easy formation of the cuff, and good maintainance of it after operation (Fig. 3).

If the cuff is not possible, we use a variant of Dudley's operation, *Pollosson's racket-like salpingostomy*: after resection of the diseased distal part, a dorsal longitudinal incision, 25 to 35 mm long is performed. The extremity is anchored to the ovary by one solid silk stitch. Then the mucosa is everted by several fine silk sutures.

The 3 last years, we have also several times performed a *bivalve variant*, which gives a well-looking fimbria, and the results are encouraging (Fig. 4).

Among 148 cases of ampullar salpingostomy, we have obtained: 75 patencies (50%), 20 U.P. (13%) and 9 U.E.P. (6%).

If we differenciate between techniques, we find:

— for the cuff: 57 cases, 25 reocclusions (43%), 32 patencies (57%), 13 U.P. (23%), 4 E.U.P. (7%).

— for the racket-type: 71 cases, 42 re-obstructions (59%) only 29 patencies (41%), 3 U.P. (4%) and 3 E.U.P. (4%).

— for the bivalve: 20 cases, 6 re-obstructions (30%), 14 patencies (70%), 4 U.P. (20%) and 2 E.U.P. (10%).

These figures suggest that the cuff and the bivalve are better that the racket, but it is necessary to stress that the last was done only when the cuff was not possible, that is in the worst cases.

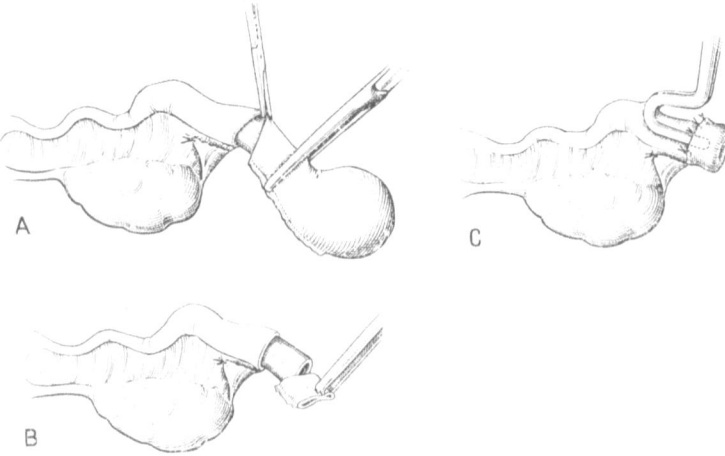

Fig. 3. Ampullar salpingostomy by the Bonney-Palmer cuff technique

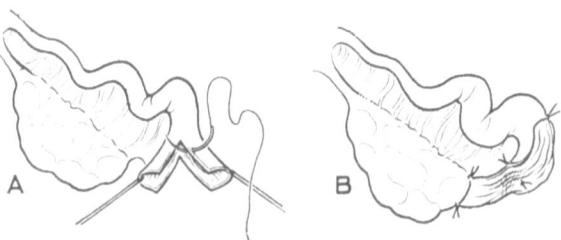

Fig. 4. Ampullar salpingostomy by the Palmer bivalve technique

Isthmic salpingostomy, either transversal or longitudinal, has never given any success in our hands in 29 cases and in most cases rapid reocclusion could be found.

An alternative to it should be subtotal linear salpingotomy, as advocated by CHA-LIER (1938).

We used this technique in 8 cases between 1938 and 1948, with three persistent patencies, and regret not to have tempted it in many cases, where we performed ovaro-uterine implantation.

Many types of prosthesis have been neggested, to avoid re-occlusion of the neo-stomy, including allantoid (GEPFERT 43) amnion (SNAITH 49) cholesterol (WESTMAN) polyethylene and silastic lubing and hoods (MULLIGAN 47, 53, 66).

Poly-ethylene tubing has never been used in our series. We have been favourably impressed by the results published with *Mulligan's silastic hoods*, claiming, in his last series of 45 cases, 81% patency, 27% U.P. and 8% E.U.P., but we have not yet used them, partly because of the necessity of a second operation after 3 months to remove the hoods.

Tubo-uterine Implantation

Tubo-uterine implantation was for us until recently the operation of choice for all proximal occlusions.

The section of the tube may be through the isthmus, or the proximal part of the ampulla. In a first period (until 1951) we advocated the ampullo-uterine implantation, because it was much more easy to carry out correctly, with a rather good rate of patencies and pregnancies. Later, we discovered some disadvantages. Most of them

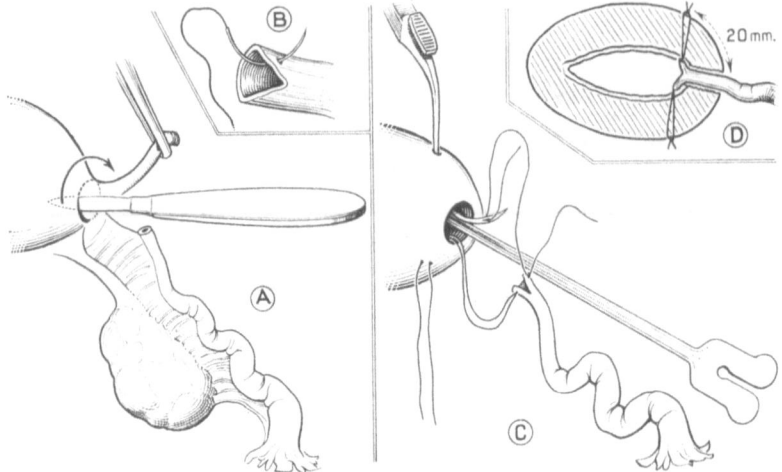

Fig. 5. Isthmo-uterine implantation by Palmer's technique

were explained by *tubal incontinence*; which might cause reflux of menstrual blood, with dysmenorrhea and sometimes secondary peri-tubal adhesions and phimosis, and even endometriosis. It was also felt that the difference between patency rate (75%) and pregnancy rate (32%) could be explained by the excessive shortening of the tube.

Therefore, mostly since 1960, we have used as often as possible the *isthmo-uterine implantation*, the isthmus being cut at first near the cornu, then, if it was too narrow, re-cut 1 cm more distally, and so on until it fits for good implantation.

Our technique is as follows (Fig. 5).

A Kocher forceps seizes the isthmus just outside the occlusion site; the tube is sectioned, and also the meso salpinx just below the tube until the uterine angle; a knife with narrow blade creates a tunnel, 5 to 7 mm of diameter, by a circular incision which, after 2 or 3 turns around the interstitial portion of the tube, penetrates the uterine cavity.

The tubal stump is then prepared for implantation: a dorsal incision 8 mm long is done on the stump, and 2 nylon 0000 stitches are put on each side of the incision at 4 mm from the angle, taking mucosa *and serosa*. Then, a grooved probe is introduced through the tunnel into the uterine cavity, and Reverdin's needle (third of circle, with a cord of 4 cm) penetrates the anterior surface of the uterus at 25 mm from the entry of the tunnel in the direction of the endometrial angle; the grooved probe is there to lead the needle toward the entry of the tunnel. The needle seizes one of the threads of the anterior flap, and then the other, by a second travel 1 mm apart from the first. Same on the posterior surface. The threads are then pulled, and the tube enters in the tunnel; they are tied cautiously (to avoid breaking) but firmly.

Our results, among 93 cases of *ampullo-uterine implantation*, are 73 patencies (78%), 31 U.P. (33%) and 8 E.U.P. (8.5%), and among 26 cases of *isthmo-uterine implantation*, performed between 1953 and 1963, are: 20 patencies (74%) 10 U.P. (43%) and 2 E.U.P. (8%).

After isthmo-uterine implantation, complete tubal incontinence is rare; in most cases, the insufflation curve is above 30 mm Hg and presents characteristic oscillations. Dysmenorrhea also is rare. Re-occlusion is a little more frequent (26% instead of 22%), but *pregnancy rate is higher* (43% instead of 33%).

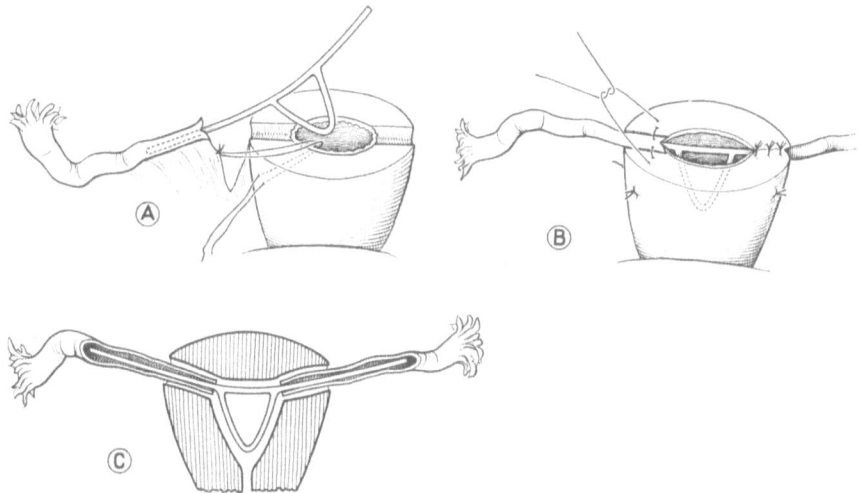

Fig. 6. Tubo-uterine implantation by Shirodkar's technique

I must confess that some collegues, after having used my technique, had re-occlusions, I feel that their failures are due to the fact that the tube was not implanted far enough so that a part of the tunnel is ready for coalescence of its walls. With the above described technique, *without poly-ethylene tubing*, the result depends entirely on the exact evaluation of the site of the endometrial angle, and the stump must really protrude a little in the uterine cavity.

Two ways to avoid the coalescence of the walls of the tunnel are possible, and may be associated:

a) One is the implantation under complete visual control — by frontal incision of the whole fundus, as advocated by SHIRODKAR, 1966.

b) The other is the use of poly-ethylene tubing, or the new Shirodkar's device (Fig. 6), but all the authors who use one or the other agree to let it stay in place at least 3 months.

In conclusion, although I still personally persist in doing implantations without intubation, I feel that the beginner in tubo-plasty should preferably use intubation or the Shirodkar's device.

Tubal Anastomosis

Tubal anastomosis, after resection of a segment of the tube, may be on the free portion of the tube or intra-mural.

Tubal anastomosis on the free portion of the tube is mostly indicated after tubal sterilization, or mid-tubal occlusions.

It is generally done with poly-ethylene tubing, and the best way to avoid expulsion of the tubing by uterine contractions, is, after a shirt median anterior hysterotomy, to insert Shirodkar's device, or to construct its equivalent with poly-ethylene tubing; four total stitches with nylon 000 are enough.

Our personal series is short: 3 cases, with 2 U.P. and 1 E.U.P.

Intra-mural anastomosis has been advocated by EHRLER (1966) as a substitute for tubal implantation, because it would avoid the risk of tubal incontinence, and preserve the true tubo-uterine junction, which seems to control the migration of the egg. He states that, in most cases of proximal occlusion, its site is not at the ostium, but 10 to 20 mm more laterally.

The indurated segment is first resected, then the uterine angle cut perpendicularly, and the interstitial tube catheterized, or visualized by retrograde hydrotubation with blue dye. If the passage is poor, the uterine angle is cut 1 or 2 more times, until good patency is evident. Then a poly-ethylene tubing is inserted in the tube and passes into the uterus through the preserved tubo-uterine junction. (A short anterior hysterotomy may help to make a ring with the intra-uterine part of the tube). The tubing be removed after 8 to 10 days.

EHRLER, among 29 personal cases, has 12 U.P. (41%) and 2 E.U.P. (6.8%), which compares favourably with the results of the implantations.

The intra-mural anastomosis is now advocated by SHIRODKAR (1968), and I have done recently two of them, and shall probably use it everytime a recent H.S.G. demonstrates a preserved normal interstitial portion of the tube.

Combined Operations on the Same Tube

Combined operations on the same tube (Implantation + Salpingostomy) may be the only solution for some cases with bipolar occlusion, if the situation has not been diagnosed before the operation through laparoscopy. I have done it in 87 private cases between 1956 and 1965, with 2 U.P. (2.2%), 4 E.U.P. (4.5%) and 46 re-occlusions (53%), most of them at the fimbria. 25 of them (29%) were latent tuberculosis; 4 of them had to submit to ulterior salpingectomy.

Some complementary operative steps

Some complementary operative steps seem to us very important in the *prevention of new adhesions*. They are:

1. *Subtotal omentectomy*, advocated by EHRLER, which we perform when the omental adhesions are extensive or dense.

2. *Uterine suspension*, mostly by the Pellanda ligamentopexy technique, to avoid postoperative retroversion and prolapse of the adnexae at the site of previous adhesions.

3. *Ovarian temporary suspension* by one stitch of catgut fixing the lateral pole of the ovary to the peritoneum of fossa iliaca, just outside the iliac artery.

4. *Perfect hemostasis* and final meticulous removal of all clots.

5. *Perfect peritonisation*, eventually with a peritoneal flap, resected from the vesico-uterine fold.

6. Any other useful operations on uterus (myomectomy, etc.) or ovaries (resection of foci of endometriosis, wedge resection for poly cystic ovary) etc. But we *avoid appendicectomy*, especially if we intend to use high dosage cortisone therapy.

Perioperative Care

Perioperative care, to suppress the normal inflammatory reaction to the surgical trauma, consists of:

a) *High dosage intra-muscular dexamethazone* (16 mg every 4 h, beginning 4 h before the operation, until the next morning), as advocated by HORNE (1966).

b) *High dosage intra-peritoneal hydrocortisone acetate* (1000 mg in 20 ml of saline, injected in the pelvic cavity, just before closing the peritoneum).

This association has been studied by SWOLIN in animal experiment and in the human, with systematical laparoscopic control 6 months after the operation.

We are using it for the last 2 years, without any trouble, and find a better patency rate, but it is too early to make definite conclusions.

We do often also a *hydrotubation on the third postoperative day* with 500 mg of hydrocortisone acetate in 20 ml of saline, in order to wash away fibrin clots which may tend to agglutinate the fimbria, and give a new dose of the drug, the action of which lasts about 4 days.

Antibiotics are given routinely for 5 days — either penicillin-streptomycin, once a day — or penicillin-colimycin, twice a day — or some other combination.

Early mobilisation is advocated by Miss MOORE-WHITE, with frequent positional modifications, to avoid the pelvic organs to stay in immobile contact.

We give *dexamethazone* per os for 3 or 4 more weeks, 6 tablets (of 0.5 mg) a day the first week, 3 tablets the next 3 weeks.

An *insufflation* is generally done 1 month after the operation, and repeated each second month, 2 or 3 times.

Control hysterosalpingography is generally done after 6 to 8 months.

Control laparoscopy is performed, if pregnancy has not occurred after 12 to 18 months; it was several times possible, at this occasion, to suppress, with the biopsy forceps of the special operative Wolf laparoscope, adhesions around the fimbria or the ovary, and 5 times a pregnancy occurred in the 3 next months.

References

Complete bibliography until 1964 may be found in MARCHESI, ALBANO, CITTADINI's book "Le Salpingoplastiche" universo editors, Rome 1965.

More recent important publications are:

HORNE, P. H.: Int. J. Fertil. **11**, 271 (1966).

MULLIGAN, W.: Int. J. Fertil. **11**, 385 (1966).

PALMER, R.: Chirurgie restauratrice tubaire dans la stérilité. Encyclopedie Medico Chirurgicale, techniques Chirurgicales. Gynécologie 41, 550—565 (1967).

—, J. DE BRUX, M. COGNAT, J. COHEN, M. GORDJI, J. NOEL et J. VINOURD: Le traitement chirurgical des stérilités tubaires. Congrès de la Fédération des Sociétés de Gynécologie et d'Obst. de langue française, Paris 1968, Bull. Fed. Soc. Gynéc. Obstet. franç. 1968.

PASETTO, N.: La Chirurgia funzionale della tuba 52. Congresso Nazionale della Società italiana di Ostetr. Ginec. Rome 1966.

SHIRODKAR, V.: Vth World Congress on Fertility, Stockholm 1966. Excerpta Medica editors, pp. 230—353.

SWOLIN, K.: Beträge zur operativen Behandlung der weiblichen Sterilität, vol. 1. Göteborg: Elanders édit. 1967.

Histopathology and Biology of Carcinoma in Situ

H. HAMPERL

"Cancer of the cervix is now regarded as a preventable disease" — so ran the statement in one of the publications of WHO (1964); a well known pathologist chimed in by saying: "We see the day ahead when there will be no more invasive carcinoma of the cervix and many of us, we hope, will live to see this day". These highflying statements, hopes and predictions are based on two assumptions:

I. Every invasive carcinoma (i. ca.) of the cervix evolves through a preparatory stage called carcinoma in situ (ca.i.s.).

II. Every ca.i.s., after some duration turns into an i.ca.; this transition can be prevented by recognition and adequate treatment of the ca.i.s.

Considering the immense practical implications of these statements it seems worth while to look closer into the evidence, on which they are based.

I.

It was a great scientific achievement, when the combined efforts of gynecologists and pathologists succeeded in establishing the following fact: in contrast to the old classical belief, that the i.ca. of the cervix originates from normal squamous epithelium, there is in many cases to be found an intermediate stage which is now generally called ca.i.s. (Table 1). It is intermediate in two aspects: clinically, as the lesion antecedes the i.ca. and morphologically, as the lesion holds a middle position between normal and cancerous epithelium.

Let us first discuss the purley histological aspects of the problem! It soon became clear that *two boundaries were difficult for the histologists to establish.*

Table 1	Table 2
Normal Epithelium	Normal Epithelium
Carcinoma in situ	Dysplasia
Invasive carcinoma	Carcinoma in situ
	Invasive carcinoma

The histological picture of the ca.i.s. is frequently not easy to separate from a lesion commonly called *dysplasia* (Table 2); this lesion in turn fades morphologically into the normal squamous epithelium. We have to admit that practically all efforts to establish a clear-cut boundary between dysplasia and ca.i.s. have failed. This statement should, however, not obscure the fact that typical cases of ca.i.s. and dysplasia are nowadays easily and uniformly diagnosed by all competent histologists. It is only the boundary-region between these two lesions, where discrepancies in the evaluation of the histological picture many occur as several tests have shown (SIEGLER, 1956; GOVAR et al., 1966; HOLMQUIST et al., 1967). I, therefore, would prefer not to put all lesions between typical ca.i.s. and normal epithelium under the heading "boundary-lesions" (KOSS et al., 1963), but to reserve this term for cases not falling unequivocally into the category of dysplasia or ca.i.s. By following this concept one can hope to reach a higher consensus between the diagnoses of different histologists.

An other area of uncertainty we encounter at the boundary between ca.i.s. and i.ca. At the first glance no diagnostic doubts seem to exist about ca.i.s. and the smallest i.ca., the microcarcinoma (Table 3). The latter shows all the histological qualities of the classic i.ca. and differs from it only by the smaller size and, therefore, remains clinically occult, as a "preclinical" carcinoma. Most characteristic is, in our opinion, the netlike arrangement of the epithelial strands infiltrating only the superficial layer of the stroma. There are, however, cases of ca.i.s. where single protrusions of the surface epithelium seem to project into the stroma. As they often show a pointed end they have been likened to the claws of a crayfish. This picture is usually to be found at many places in a given case of ca.i.s. and is known as *"early stromal invasion"* (FENNELL, 1955; FRIEDELL et al., 1958) — with the silent understanding that a "late stromal invasion" would already be a (micro-)invasive ca. Many authors do not

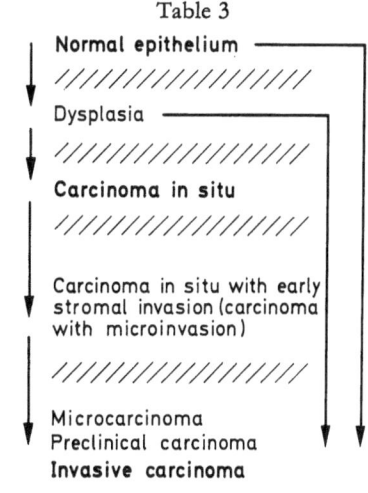

Table 3

hesitate to put the diagnosis "carcinoma" on this picture although with the complementing adjectiv "micro-invasive" or "superficially invasive" (DILWORTH and MAXWELL, 1962). They regard the destruction of the basal membrane as evidence for

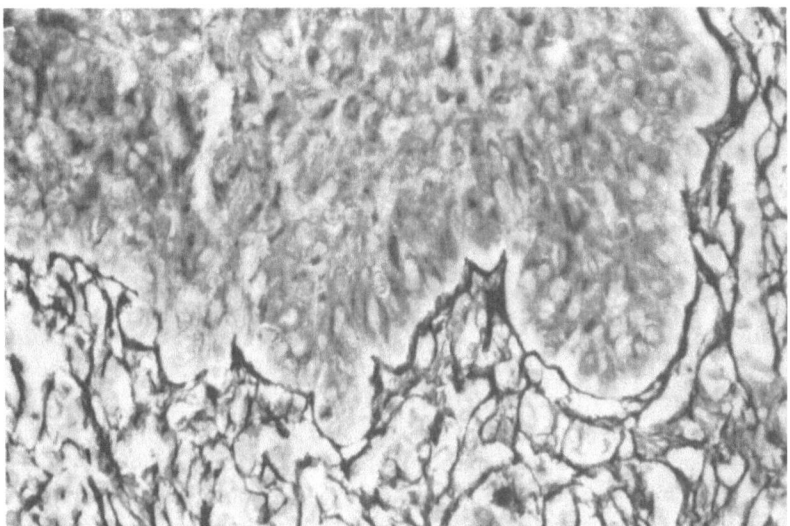

Fig. 1. Ca.i.s. with beginning stromal invasion. The basal membrane not interrupted but pushed downwards. Reticulin-stain with silver. (From HAMPERL, 1966)

malignancy. By systematically studying this "microinvasion" I found (1966) that it may proceed in two ways; either the intact basal membrane is pushed downwards and accompanies the epithelial outgrowth as an uninterrupted layer (Fig. 1 u. 3/I), or the basal membrane is disappearing through the action of invading migrant cells, predominantly lymphocytes (Fig. 3/IIa). The epithelium then only uses these breaks to grow into the stroma (Fig. 2 u. 3/IIb) but does not by itself produce the breaks in the basal membrane.

As one can see not only the boundary between ca.i.s. and dysplasia but also between ca.i.s. and i.ca. seems to be somewhat blurred, depending upon whether we put a lesion with early stromal invasion (microinvasion) into the category of ca.i.s. or microcarcinoma. Generally the latter is done in order to be on the safe side when treating patient. The question is however not finally settled from the point of view of the pathologist. For him it is only clear, that there is a very strict biological dividing-line between all kind of precancerous lesions and real cancer as manifested by a

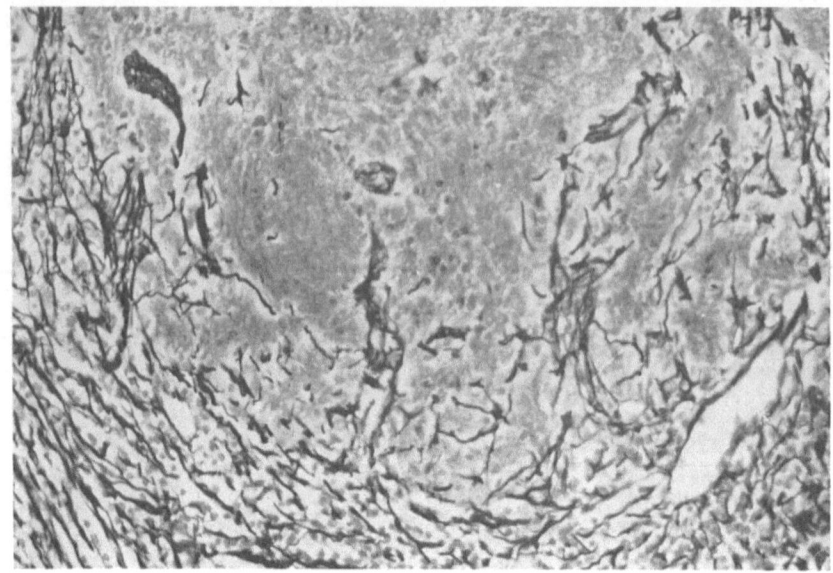

Fig. 2. Ca.i.s. with early stromal invasion. The epithelial masses growing downwards into the spaces between the reticulin fibers. Reticulin-stain with silver. (From HAMPERL, 1966)

fundamentally different pattern of chromosomes, grade of ploidy and DNA-content of the nuclei (KIRKLAND et al., 1967; AUERSPERG et al., 1967).

Finally, some *subdivisions* have been suggested even *in the area of unquestionable ca.i.s.* (Table 4). There are cases where the epithelium of the ca.i.s. simply replaces the normal epithelium on the surface (Fig. 4), in others the pathological epithelium is extending downwards into the cervical glands or clefts (Fig. 4), displacing and replacing the normal cylindrical epithelium, and finally converting the gland into a solid epithelial mass by entirely filling the lumen. As pointed out by HILLEMANNS (1964, 1968) another variety is due to the fact that the epithelium sometimes pushes downwards into the stroma through bulky outgrowth (Fig. 5) sometimes accompanied by a crowding of cells. The same author regards areas of cellmaturation either located inside the surface epithelium or peripherally towards the stroma as a special sign of impending infiltration. Many other authors including myself (1959) have tried to classify ca.i.s. into subgroups (NESBITT and STEIN, 1958; FLUHMANN, 1960; NIEBURGS, 1963; TITKIN, 1963; BURGHARDT, 1964; ATKIN, 1964; OLD et al., 1965;

WIELENGA et al., 1965) but none of these classifications has till now been generally accepted.

It is very tempting to arrange all these somehow related pictures into a row, and by so doing, succumb to the very suggestive assumption that they represent not

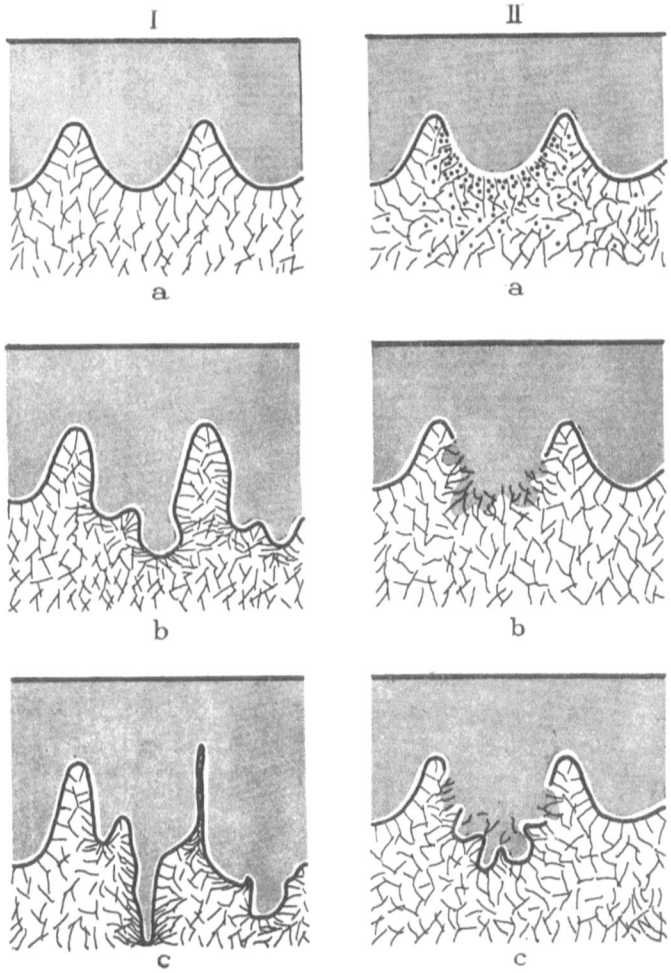

Fig. 3. The different behaviour of the basal membrane and the reticulin fibers in ca.i.s. (grey). I/a—c: The intact basal membrane is pushed downwards as in Fig. 1; II/a: The basal membrane is dissolved while lymphocytes emigrate; II/b: The ca.i.s. uses these breaks to infiltrate into the spaces between the reticulin fibers as in Fig. 2; II/c: At some places a new basal membrane is formed. (From HAMPERL, 1966)

Table 4. *Carcinoma in situ*

Symply replacing normal epithelium
Infiltrating cervical glands
Preinvasive crowding of cells (bulky outgrowth)
With intraepithelial areas of maturation
Large-cell type
Small-cell type

merely a pathohistologic fiction but the natural course of events leading eventually to i.ca. (Table 3, arrows at left). There are in fact some indications that this may be so: HERTIG, FIDLER and BOYD (1960), DUNN and PURVIS (1967) and others, pointed to the different age groups affected by the different lesions: the dysplasia and ca.i.s.

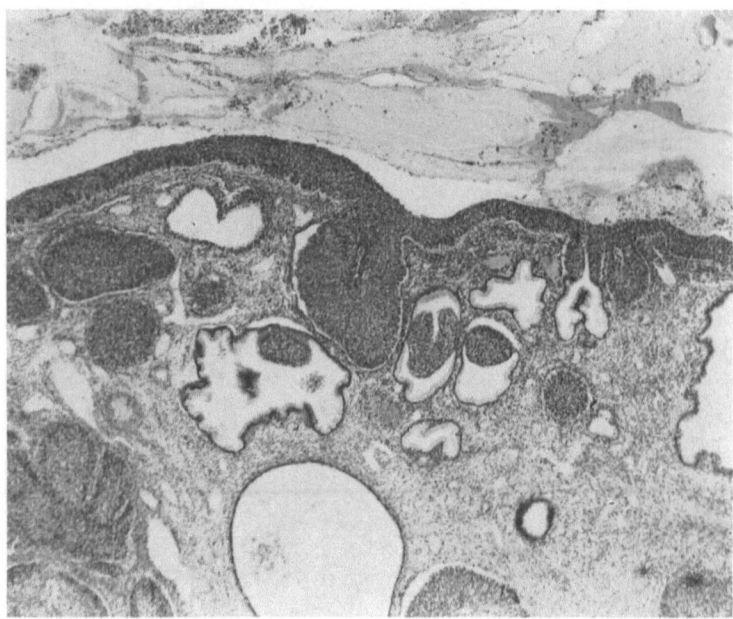

Fig. 4. Ca.i.s. with simple replacing growth on the surface and filling the lumina of the cervical glands

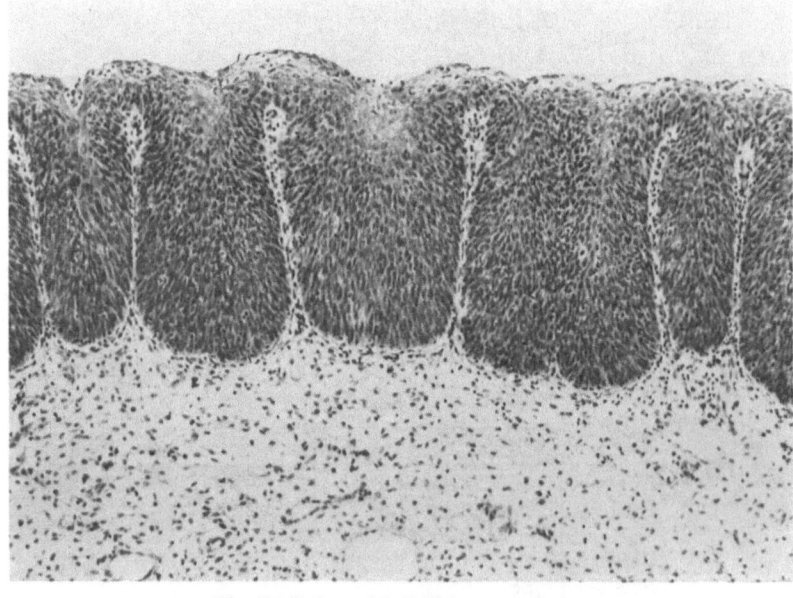

Fig. 5. Ca.i.s. with bulky outgrowth

occuring at a younger age than the i.ca. It was even calculated that ca.i.s. needed an average of 5 to 8 years in order to progress to an i.ca. The strongest argument in favor of the theory of a slow progression from bad to worse came from the clinical observation of untreated cases of ca.i.s. developing into i.ca. after several years duration.

It remains, however, still questionable whether in these cases the progression runs through all the histological patterns so neatly arranged by the pathologist. There exist, indeed, several reports indicating other possibilities (Table 3, arrows at right): BURGHARDT (1967) has recently published four cases, in which he felt reasonably sure that an i.ca. developed immediately from/or in a normal epithelium; SCHILLER et al., spoke of a "spray-carcinoma" as early as 1953; in screening programs cases have turned up where there was only evidence of a previous dysplasia and not of ca.i.s., before the appearance of i.ca. (Koss et al., 1963; BANGLE et al., 1963; DUNN and PURVIS, 1967).

It seems even doubtful whether the "microinvasion" ever develops into real i.ca., since the microinvasion occurs at many places in a given ca.i.s., where as the i.ca., also in its microcarcinoma-form originates at only one definite spot (FENNELL, 1954).

On the basis of all the known facts we may, therefore, formulate the answer to our first question, whether every i.ca. of the cervix is preceeded by a ca.i.s.: *many, probably even the majority of i.ca., develop from a precancerous lesion, the ca.i.s., but by no means all of them.*

II.

The second question, whether every ca.i.s. eventually progresses into i.ca., is almost equally important from the point of view of prevention of i.ca. The problem consists in establishing to what extent the ca.i.s. is a progredient, or a stationary lesion, or even is able to regress completely. The differences in the answers in the current literature are mainly due to the lack of a clear distinction between ca.i.s. and i.ca. on one hand and dysplasia on the other, as explained earlier. If one includes in ones classification of ca.i.s. lesions, another pathologist would rather diagnose as dysplasias, one would quite correctly come to the conclusion that regression is possible. On the other hand, a narrower definition of the term ca.i.s. may lead to just the opposite conclusion.

The simple way of establishing the presence of a ca.i.s. in one of its forms and then waiting to see what happens is, unfortunately, not feasible because the inflammatory reaction following a diagnstic excision of a ca.i.s. is able to destroy the remaining parts of the lesion. The problem amounts to the impossibility of having ones cake and eating it at the same time. To rely only on cytologic evidence is open to criticism, since the method, the achievements of the cytologists not withstanding, is scarcely able to distinguish between the whole spectrum of the pertaining lesions with desirable accuracy. There are, however, cases on record with the cytological findings of ca.i.s. over many years, even decades, without any inclination towards i.ca. We can, therefore, only assume that the possibility of regression of a ca.i.s. most probably diminishes as it approaches the i.ca. BURGHARDT (1966) tried to illustrate this in a schematic drawing (Fig. 6). We, therefore, may answer our second question by the statement that *a part of the ca.i.s. in a strict sense may inevitably progress into i.ca., but by no means all ca.i.s.*

It would be of paramount interest to know how big this part is. KIRKLAND et al. (1967) think that only half or one third of all preinvasive lesions reach the stage of i.ca. Boyes et al. (1964) came on the basis of their mass-screening to the conclusion that only about 60% of all ca.i.s. become eventually i.ca. Meyer (1965) found even in about barely $1/10$ of all cases of early i.ca. (including microcarcinoma) traces of ca.i.s. Also on statistical grounds it is improbable that all ca.i.s. would progress into i.ca., as too many ca.i.s. were found compared with the lower incidence of i.ca.

As you see my answer to both initial questions is not a simple "yes" or "no" due to the fact that i.ca. may arise without a preceding ca.i.s. and a ca.i.s. may remain stationary or even regress and never develop into an i.ca. Unfortunately, even after examining our cytological and histological preparations, we are not able at present, to say exactly how frequently this occurs or when the point of no return is reached. A screening program embracing a whole population may succeed in early recognizing and consecutively weeding out all ca.i.s., but if not all these lesions would have progressed into cancer the whole action may seem, at least partly, a very costly luxury,

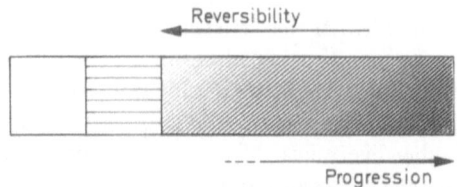

Fig. 6. The decreasing reversibility of ca.i.s. as it approaches invasiveness (right hand end of the drawing: normal epithelium at left). (From Burghardt, 1964)

the more so if i.ca. may be able to evade the screening by hiding in the cervical canal or by developing rapidly without previous warning. The real test for the usefullness of mass screening will, therefore, be a significant lowering of the death rate of i.ca. of the cervix. The pertinent statistics are still controversial in this respect (see Green, 1966) to say the least. Let us, however, hope that the optimistic statements I mention ed at the beginning of my exposé may be supported by solid facts in the future.

References

Atkin, N. B.: Nature (Lond.) **202**, 201 (1964).
Auersperg, N., M. J. Corey, and A. Worth: Cancer Res. **27**, 1394—1401 (1967).
Bangle, R., Jr., M. Berger, and M. Levin: Cancer (Philad.) **16**, 1151—1159 (1963).
Boyes, D. A., H. K. Fidler, and D. R. Lock: Brit. med. J. **1962** I, 203—205.
Burghardt, E.: Verh. dtsch. Ges. Path. **1964**, 12—33.
— Geburth. u. Frauenheilk. **27**, 1170—1180 (1967).
Dilworth, E. E., and G. E. Maxwell: Amer. J. Obstet. Gynec. **84**, 83—88 (1962).
Dunn, J. E. M., and L. Purvis: Cancer (Philad.) **20**, 1899—1906 (1967).
Fennell, R. H.: Amer. J. Path. **3**, No. 178, 623—624 (1954).
Fennell, R. F., Jr.: Cancer (Philad.) **8**, 302—309 (1955).
Fidler, H. K., and J. R. Boyd: Cancer (Philad.) **13**, 764—771 (1960).
Fluhmann, C. F.: Amer. J. Obstet. Gynec. **16**, 424—437 (1960).
Friedell, G. J., A. T. Hertig, and P. A. Younge: Arch. Path. **66**, 494—503 (1958).
Govan, A. D. T., R. M. Haines, F. A. Langley, C. W. Taylor, and A. S. Woodcock: J. Obstet. Gynaec. Brit. Cwlth, N.S. **73**, 883—896 (1966).
Green, G. H.: Amer. J. Obstet. Gynec. **94**, 1009—1022 (1966).
Hamperl, H.: Virchows Arch. path. Anat. **340**, 185—205 (1966).
— Definition and classification of the socalled carcinoma in situ. Symposium CIBA Founda tion study group No. 3:2. London: Churchill 1959.
Hillemanns, H. G.: Arch. Gynäk. **191**, 235—270 (1958).
— Entstehung und Wachstum des Zervixkarzinoms. Basel/New York: S. Karger 1964.

—, B. Sixtus-Klug und E. Prestel: Arch. Gynäk. **206**, 82—97 (1968).
Holmquist, N. D., C. A. McMahan, and O. D. Williams: Arch. Path. **84**, 334—345 (1967).
Kirkland, J. A., M. A. Stanley, and M. K. Cellier: Cancer (Philad.) **20**, 1934—1952 (1967).
Koss, L. G., F. W. Steward, F. W. Foote, M. J. Jordan, G. M. Bader, and E. Day: Cancer (Philad.) **16**, 1160—1210 (1963).
Meyer, P. C.: J. clin. Path. **18**, 414—423 (1965).
Nesbitt, R. E. L., Jr., and A. A. Stein: Surg. Gynec. Obstet. **107**, 161—168 (1958).
Nieburgs, H. E.: Cancer (Philad.) **16**, No. 2, 141—159 (1963).
Old, J. W., G. Wielenga, and E. v. Haam: Cancer (Philad.) **18**, 1598—1611 (1965).
Schiller, W., A. F. Daro, H. A. Gollin, and N. P. Primiario: Amer. J. Obstet. Gynec. **65**, 1088—1098 (1953).
Siegler, E. E.: Cancer (Philad.) **9**, 463—469 (1956).
Titkin, K. D.: Acta Un. int. Cancer **19**, 1377—1378 (1963).
Wielenga, G., J. W. Old, and E. v. Haam: Cancer (Philad.) **18**, 1612—1621 (1965).
World Health Organization: Technical Report Series Nr. 276, 1964.

Early Detection and Cytology of Carcinoma in Situ*

Günther Kern

Great numbers of the so called carcinoma in situ have been detected by cyto-diagnosis of exfoliated cells of the cervix uteri. With increasing experience the intra-epithelial malignant lesion was no longer understood as real cancer, but as a pre-cancerous lesion, which precedes cervical cancer.

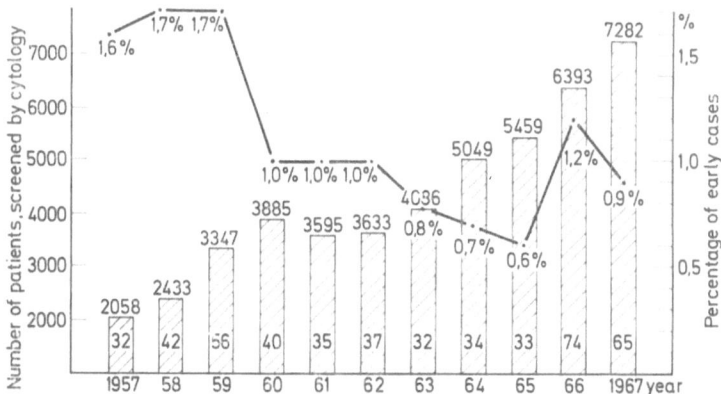

Fig. 1. Results of the cytologic examination of 47220 women. 480 (1.02%) early cases have been detected. (Dysplasia: 67, carcinoma in situ: 364, microcarcinoma: 49)

The clinical consequence was the limitation of the therapeutical approach. Today the excision of the area concerned the so called conization is the method of choice.

Younge in 1957 expressed the opinion, that cervical cancer is a preventable disease, if every women had adequate precautious examinations. The World Health Organization recently also came to the same opinion. Before discussing the part of cytology in reaching this objective, I should like to point out some important aspects in our experience with the cytodiagnosis of carcinoma in situ.

* From the University Hospital of Gynecology and Obstetrics Cologne (Direktor: Prof. Dr. C. Kaufmann).

555

1. Without doubt the detection of premalignant epithelial atypias is most successfully accomplished by means of cytology. The carcinoma in situ is neither detectable
by inspection with the naked eye, nor by gynecological palpation. The inspection of

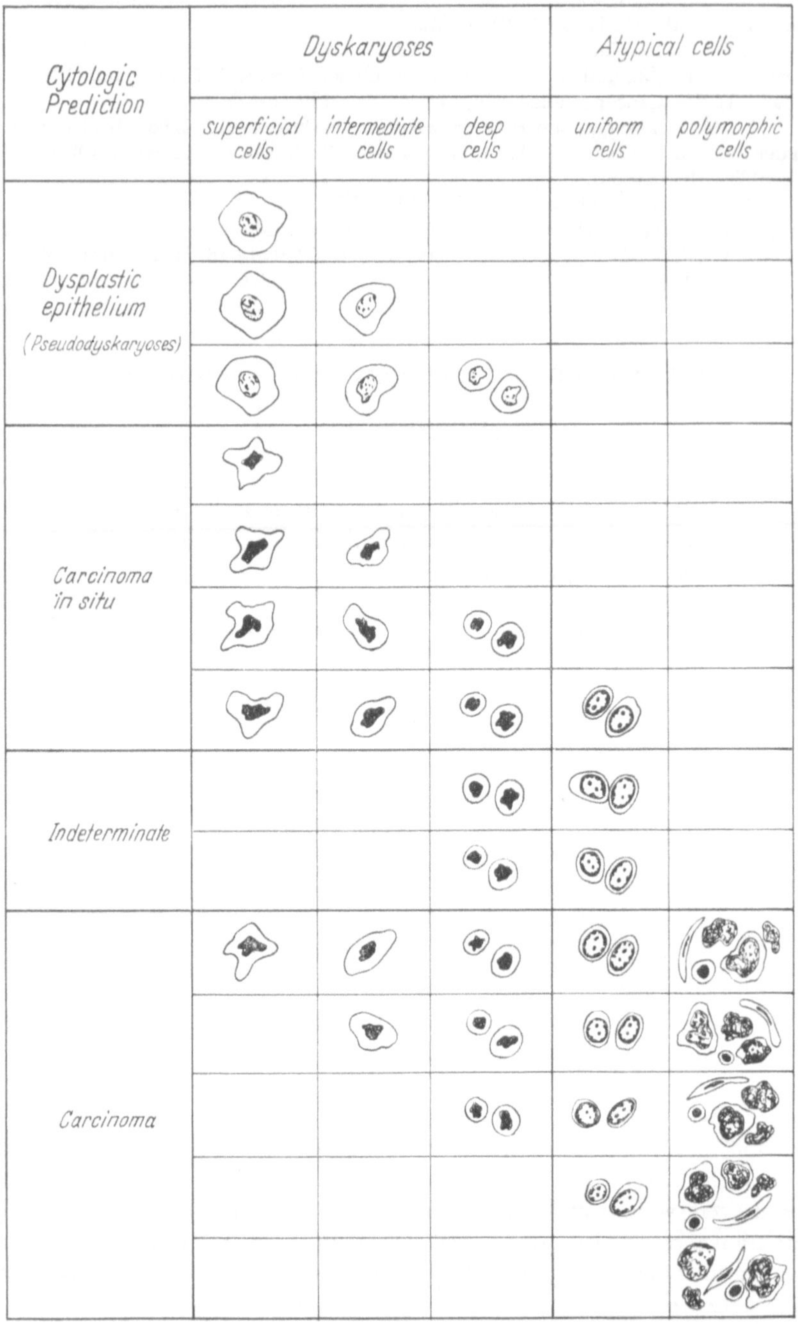

Fig. 2. Partly schematic representation of cellular types in the cytologic smear, from which
a prediction can be made about the histologic change. (KERN, 1962)

the cervical surface with a magnifying glass called colposcopy also has many disadvantages in comparison with cytology. Fig. 1 shows the number of patients examined cytologically in the past 11 years as well as the numbers and percentages of the detected and treated early cases. We investigated 47220 mostly out-patients in the University Hospital of Gynecology and Obstetrics in Cologne.

We found 480, this means 1.02% carcinoma in situ. This figure does not include cytologically detected but clinically still asymptomatic invasive cancers. Mass-screening programs of presumably healthy women usually arrive at a percentage of around 0.5.

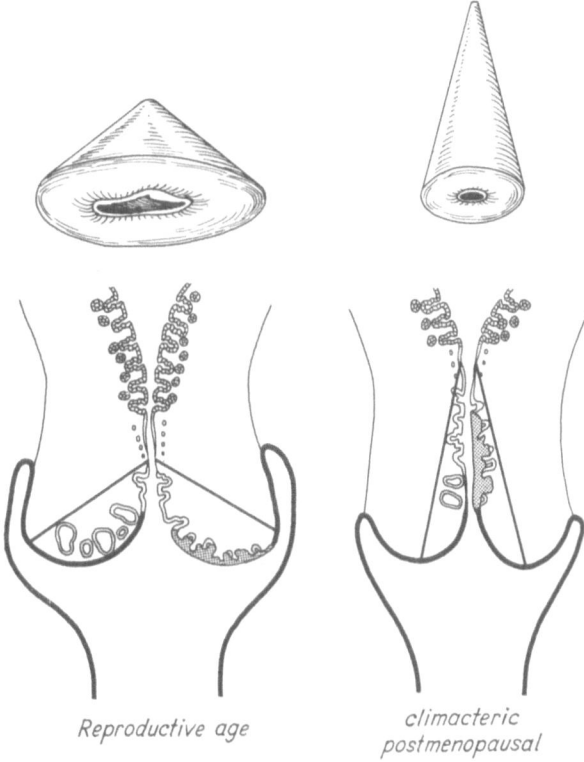

Reproductive age

climacteric
postmenopausal

Fig. 3. Direction of incision and shapes of the cones of tissue by cervical conization, depending on the patient's age. (Modified after OBER and BÖTZELEN, 1959)

2. Because of the close collaboration with histology lasting for many years we have been able to correlate the cytological picture with the histological lesion (Fig. 2).

From the appearance of certain cell-types in the cytological smear, which I cannot discuss in detail in this presentation we reach a prediction of the histological epithelial atypia with an accuracy of around 90%. For the clinician the cytological prediction has the following consequences: If the smear indicates a dysplasia, the patient is scheduled for cytological controls in regular intervals. A treatment is not yet indicated. If the cytological prediction indicates a carcinoma in situ, or — in a very small group — a prediction is not possible, the patient is diagnosed and treated by conization in one procedure (Fig. 3). In elderly women we also consider a hysterectomy. If so called polymorphic atypical cells appear in the smear our experience indicates an invasive cancer. After the usual methods of biopsies the patient is treated by radical operation or radiationtherapy. The presentation of Prof. HAMPERL has shown, that the transition between dysplasia and carcinoma in situ in the same case may be not well defined. But also histologically it may be difficult to decide, if one still deals with a dysplasia or already with a carcinoma in situ. It is obvious that this kind of diagnosis is even more difficult from single cells in the smear no longer in contact with the epithelium.

I stress this point, because internationally a variable diagnostic value is attached to both lesions. Therefore some doubts were recently expressed about the biological significance of carcinoma in situ as a precancerous lesion.

Results of prospective cytology	Number of cases	%	Observation time → histologic diagnosis	Type of histologic change
Stationary	6	(7.4)	3—5 years	Dysplasia
	16	(19.8)	2—8 years	Carcinoma in situ
Progression normal → Dysplasia → carcinoma in situ	30	(37.0)	2—9 years	Carcinoma in situ
normal → dysplacia → carcinoma in situ → invasive carcinoma	3	(3.7)	4—9 years	invasive cancer
Regression Dysplasia → normal	26	(32.1)	2—11 years (Cytological observation time)	normal epithelium (only six patients had a curettage)
	81	(100.0)		

Fig. 4. Long period observations with prospective cytology

3. As I already mentioned, we do not treat but control patients with a dysplasia. Women with more severe lesions are always scheduled for treatment. Nevertheless 81 patients during 11 years declined treatment, but they came for cytological controls. In this cases we could do long-term observation by means of prospective cytology. We investigated whether the lesion behaved stationary, progressive or regressive, without having been able to disturb the development of the lesion by biopsies.

It was first pointed out by PAPANICOLAOU in 1949 that only observation-periods with the smear method may give an answer about the development of intraepithelial changes, because any kind of biopsy may excise totally, or damage or miss the lesion. Fig. 4 gives a general survey about the 81 cases. In 22 patients the cytological smears were *stationary* and did not change within 2 to 8 years indicating a dysplasia or a carcinoma in situ. The observation time was terminated with the treatment of the patient. However the beginning of the epithelial atypia is still unknown.

33 patients showed a *progression* within 2 to 9 years. The cytological smears had been unsuspicious for several months and changed afterwards to dysplasia or carcinoma in situ. Of special interest are three patients, where the step to the invasive cancer could exactly be recognized in the cytological smears. Fig. 5 shows an example. The third group behaved *regressively*, that means, the pathological celltypes could be recognized for several months up to 3 and 4 years and disappeared afterwards. In this group it is of special importance that we observed a regression only in those cases, which indicated cytologically a dysplasia. In women with cytological findings indicating a carcinoma in situ we never found a regressive tendency.

I should like to summarize briefly:

1. Premalignant epithelial atypies at the cervix uteri are best detected by means of cytology.

2. It is possible to correlate the cytological picture with the histological lesion.

3. Long-term-observation periods demonstrated, that a carcinoma in situ may be stationary over many years. Our material shows in no case a tendency of regression.

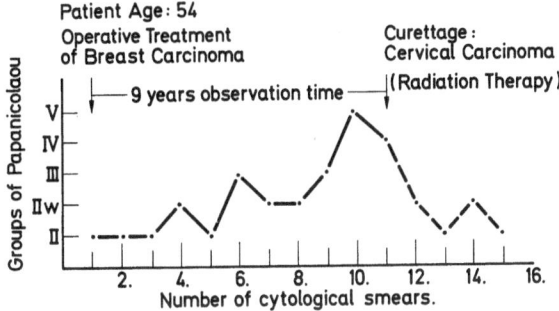

Fig. 5. Cell types in the smears changed from normal cells up to polymorphic tumor cells over a period of 9 years. In this patient a progression of the epithelial atypia could be observed by means of cytology

However dysplasia may be regressive in a very high percentage. The step from carcinoma in situ to invasive cancer seems to proceed rather quickly.

May I finally come back to the question whether we have reached the objective of preventing cervical cancer.

Unfortunately this aim still is far away. Countries with a high population are only able to screen a very small percentage of all females. In Cologne, which has a very good screening program, we estimate that it includes about 10% of all women in 1 year. If a higher percentage took part in, we would not have enough cytologically trained people, to examine such mass-material. An excessive work load for the doctors and technicians and other factors would lead to an increase of false negative cytological results, which would give the patients a false feeling of security. If a women returns to a cytological examination in yearly intervals in 1 to 2% a precancerous lesion may be detected and in some cases even an invasive cancer.

The cytodiagnosis of the cervix uteri is the most reliable method to recognize premalignant lesions. However, a significant prevention of cervical cancer has not yet been achieved despite all efforts.

Surgical Treatment of Carcinoma in Situ of the Cervix Uteri*

Woodard D. Beacham, and Edwin Hugh Lawson Jr.

At the Congress of the International Federation of Gynecology and Obstetrics held in Vienna in 1961 the Cancer Committee under the chairmanship of Kottmeier defined stage 0, carcinoma of the cervix as preinvasive carcinoma, so-called carcinoma in situ. In 1964 the American College of Obstetricians and Gynecologists distributed *Clinical Staging System for Carcinoma of the Cervix* by the American Joint Committee for Cancer Staging and End Results Reporting. This Committee is sponsored by the American College of Surgeons, the American College of Radiology, the College of American Pathologists, the American College of Physicians, the American Cancer Society, and the National Cancer Institute. The brochure contained the above definition and designated the clinical stage as TO carcinoma in situ (intraepithelial). Its detection and eradication offer marvelous opportunity to prevent the havoc caused by invasive cancer. The advantages of treating any disease in its asymptomatic state is obvious.

In 1965 Hamperl [1965 (1)] discussed what is meant by the term "carcinoma in situ". In the same year he [1965 (2)] described the prestages and early stages of cervical carcinoma.

In an editorial in the February 1968 issue of *Obstetrics and Gynecology* Demin of the Cancer Unit of WHO discusses "some aspects of carcinoma in situ of the uterine cervix". He presents various viewpoints hoping "to provoke more discussions on this important subject and to obtain views and guidance to clarify the definition, limits, and proper use of this term of so great importance to pathologists, gynecologists, and oncologists". Green has presented his views regarding the significance of cervical carcinoma in situ which are at variance to those generally held by contributors to the literature. Ashley thinks there is strong evidence for the existence of two forms of cervical carcinoma. Jones et al. used a direct squash technic to study the chromosomes of tissue from the cervix from patients with atypia, carcinoma in situ, and invasive epidermoid carcinoma of the cervix. They concluded: "The findings are not inconsistent with the concept that aneuploidy is concurrent with cancer, but further study will be required to unequivocally establish this possibility and to demonstrate the diagnostic role of chromosome determination in early cancer of the cervix". At the recent meeting of the American Gynecological Society his subject was "The Value of the Assay of Chromosomes in the Diagnosis of Neoplasia". An abstract of his dissertation is as follows: "It now seems well established that most invasive epidermoid carcinomas and intraepithelial carcinomas of the cervix are composed of cells displaying aneuploidy. In lesions which are less severe than unequivocal carcinoma, it is important to determine when cytogenetic abnormalities first appear in relation to abnormalities revealed by other diagnostic methods, such as colposcopy, cytopathology and histopathology. The present study correlates the assay of chromosomes with findings of other diagnostic studies on more than 20 patients with early cervical neoplasia. From these data an estimate may be made of the value of karyotype analysis in the management of patients with squamous atypia of the cervix".

* From the Department of Obstetrics and Gynecology, Tulane University School of Medicine, Tulane Unit, Charity Hospital of Louisiana at New Orleans, and Southern Baptist Hospital, New Orleans.

68 years ago CULLEN's monograph on Cancer of the Uterus appeared. 8 years later SCHAUENSTEIN published his histologic studies of the cervix. 2 years threeafter RUBIN wrote on the pathological diagnosis of incipient carcinoma of the uterus. This was followed by SCHOTTLANDER and KERMAUNER's volume *Zur Kenntnis des Uterus-carcinoms*. To MEYER and SCHILLER must go credit in the recognition of the work on carcinoma in situ of the cervix. HINSELMANN's classic article in *Zbl. Gynäk.* appeared in 1927. The popularity of the colposcope in European clinics resulted in frequent cervical biopsy and study of cervical lesions earlier than in the United States of America. However, it must be said that PEMBERTON and SMITH reported their series under the title of the early diagnosis and prevention of carcinoma of the cervix in 1929. In 1928 at the Third Race Betterment Conference PAPANICOLAOU presented "new cancer diagnosis through the recognition of exfoliated cancer cells". 5 years later SCHILLER wrote in the Official Scientific Journal of the American College of Surgeons on the early diagnosis of carcinoma of the cervix. In 1943 the volume entitled *Diagnosis of Uterine Cancer by the Vaginal Smear* by PAPANICOLAOU and TRAUT resulted in the acceptance and appreciation of this excellent diagnostic procedure. DOUGLAS informs us that PAPANICOLAOU graduated at the University of Athens Medical School and went to Vienna to study philosophy. Disenchantment followed and he enrolled at Hertig's Institute for Experimental Biology at the University of Munich. In 1949 YOUNGE et al. reported 135 cases of carcinoma in situ. Since then substantial series have been reported by those authors shown in Table 1 and others. In 1963 FUNNELL and MERRILL reported a recurrence rate of 8.1% in 74 cases. Published tables compiled from reported cases regarding vaginal recurrencies and/or invasive carcinoma must be analyzed taking into consideration the thoroughness of the surgical procedure in each case, the total number of patients treated, and the time interval since treatment. Undoubtedly there have been cases in which areas of carcinoma in situ in the upper vagina have not been excised. Some so-called "recurrences" are attributable to field cancerization for embryologic reasons. Others are explainable by the multicentric origin of cancer in the genital tract. The reader is referred to articles by MARCUS, NEWMAN and CROMER, HALLGRIMISSON, LAUCHLAN, and STAHMANN.

It would probably be startlingly interesting to know the number of women whose cervical carcinoma in situ has been cured by postpartum electric cauterization. The senior author has been and continues to be a strong advocate of the procedure in cases where there are eversions, erosions and/or cysts provided PAPANICOLAOU smears are negative.

Given a patient with a proved diagnosis of carcinoma in situ of the cervix one must consider the following. Is she pregnant? If so, what is the duration of gestation? What are her age, gravidity, parity, and number of living children? Does she desire additional progeny? What is her general condition? What signs and symptoms are present or elicitable? What is her attitude toward her uterus? What is her husband's attitude toward it? Time explaining the function of the uterus may prevent unhappiness to all concerned. Ignorance causes uncertainty. In *Maxims in Prose* JOHANN WOLFGANG GOETHE said, "What we do not understand we do not possess".

In surgically treating each patient it is essential to individualize the patient. She must not be treated as a statistic.

It is generally agreed that if a cervical lesion is present, punch biopsy is indicated. TE LINDE and others have been strong advocates of multiple punch biopsies. If this procedure reveals some condition less severe than invasive carcinoma or the cervix presents a homogeneous appearance, multiple sections must be examined by the pathologist so that he can properly report on the condition of the cervix. Most of the workers agree that this is best accomplished by submitting a cold knife cone specimen to the pathologist. If his final analysis confirms the presence of cervical carcinoma in situ the definitive treatment recommended is total hysterectomy with adequate excision of the vaginal cuff. The type of hysterectomy will depend upon the case. Inasmuch as patients with carcinoma in situ frequently present a history of multiparity and findings of pelvic relaxation, hysterectomy is often performed by the vaginal route with the indicated reparative procedures.

Writing on the evaluation of biopsy, cone and hysterectomy sequence in intraepithelial carcinoma of the cervix SILBAR and WOODRUFF stated: "In a series of 124 cases in which biopsy, cone and hysterectomy specimens were available, there were three instances in which invasive cervical cancer was not discovered on biopsy but recognized in the cone, an incidence of 2.4%. In an additional 61 cases, 8 instances of invasive carcinoma were not recognized in biopsy material but discovered in the cone specimen. The overall error in the 195 cases was 5.94%. Biopsy is an important step in the planned diagnostic study of cervical disease. It is imperative that the biopsy be adequate and that the pathologist's report include a statement as to its adequacy. The more widespread use of such diagnostic tools as colposcopy in association with the directed biopsy...may lead to refinement in diagnosis of cervical disease and reduction in percentage error in tissue study".

If childbearing function is to be preserved, cervical conization is the treatment advised. If that operation reveals no evidence of invasion, the patient is seen for examination and PAPANICOLAOU smears every 3 months for 1 year and every 6 months thereafter. If the cervical and vaginal smears continue to be normal the patient is advised to become pregnant. If the smears again show cytologic abnormality further investigation is indicated and definitive therapy may be necessary. If the smear during pregnancy indicates the necessity for re-evaluation and it is necessary to perform a cervical conization to rule out invasive carcinoma, it is advised that the procedure be done during the second trimester of pregnancy. If only carcinoma in situ is proved by conization during pregnancy the patient should be allowed to deliver vaginally unless there are obstetric indications for cesarean section.

Cervical Conization

In 1955 SCHIFFER et al. reported 210 cervical conizations. In a discussion of their technic they mention that a 1:100,000 Neosynephrine solution is injected submucosally and into the body of the cervix. In their summary they state: "The extended cone biopsy may be used as the definitive treatment for carcinoma in situ in selected patients. Cytologic follow-up of patients having had this procedure is an intrinsic part of the procedure".

In 1960 HESTER and READ evaluated 155 cervical conizations listing the indications and complications. They stressed the reliability of this procedure for diagnostic purposes. They concluded: "The high percentage of residual abnormal cervical epithelium in the uterus following conization re-emphasizes total hysterectomy as the treatment of choice in carcinoma in situ".

At the 1966 meeting of the Central Association of Obstetricians and Gynecologists ROGERS and WILLIAMS evaluated the impact of the suspicious PAPANICOLAOU smear on the outcome of pregnancy. They stated: "102 pregnant patients who were found to have suspicious smears were studied. Over 40% were found to have carcinoma in situ but none had frank invasive carcinoma. Of the patients subjected to conization, $1/3$ had postoperative complications. There were significant and related perinatal problems in approximately $1/5$. The immediate routine conization biopsy when the repeated suspicious PAPANICOLAOU smear is found in a pregnant patient is a rule of therapy which should be challenged, studied, and revised. This conclusion is at odds with the opinions of a majority of the chiefs of approved Obstetrics and Gynecology residency programs whose views were surveyed." This was a study of nationwide attitudes and maternal and perinatal complications.

In 1967 ANDERSON and LINTON presented the results of a retrospective survey of 415 cervical conizations comparing the diagnostic accuracy of cervical biopsy and cervical conizations. They wrote: "Conization of the cervix is recommended as the diagnostic procedure of choice after an abnormal cytologic smear because of its greater accuracy."

In 1967 ADELMAN and HAJDU reviewed a series of 100 cone biopsy specimens diagnosed as carcinoma in situ followed by hysterectomy. They stated: "The purpose of the study was to determine when the cone biopsy in itself may constitute the final therapy for carcinoma in situ. The data, although statistically insignificant, suggest that such a predictable relationship does exist and that hysterectomy can be bypassed in certain patients provided that a close follow-up is assured." They concluded: "An undeniable risk is associated with conservative therapy of carcinoma in situ and this must be weighed against the equally undeniable risk associated with overtreatment to determine the proper course of action in individual patients."

In 1968 CRISP et al. discussed shallow conization of the cervix, having performed it in 232 patients for diagnostic purposes. They found carcinoma in 41% of the specimens. The chief advantage of the method is the relative freedom from complications. In a discussion of their technic they mention the use of Ioprep[1]. They stated that this stains the cervix like Schiller's solution. They suggest the use of scissors after the incision is carried around the circumference of the cervical os to a depth of approximately 1.5 to 2 cm. After removal of the cone with the scissors the cervical canal is dilated and a fractional curettage is done. A Surgicel[2] pack is placed in the conization site. Only 4 of 227 nonpregnant patients required later suturing of the cervix according to their report.

At the 1967 meeting of District VII of the American College of Obstetricians and Gynecologists McCANN et al. presented their analysis of the records of all patients undergoing sharp conization on the Louisiana State University Unit at Charity Hospital in New Orleans from January 1, 1949 through 1964. During that time there were 431 conizations performed on 400 patients. There were no conization operative deaths or hysterectomies required for control of bleeding. Of the 114 patients with diagnosis of carcinoma in situ in the conization specimen, 29 had residual carcinoma in situ in the hysterectomy specimen.

Obviously, a candidate for cervical conization is entitled to complete preoperative evaluation. It is mandatory that she not have any disturbances in her bleeding and coagulation mechanisms. The type of anesthesia will be selected in each case. Although FLEMING and others have devised special conization instruments the use of the scalpel

---

[1] Arbrook, Somerville, N.J.
[2] Surgicel, Johnson & Johnson, New Brunswick, N.J.

blade is most common. Over 20 years ago CROSSEN advocated extensive conization using an electrode but this method had a destructive effect on the tissues to be examined. Technics for cervical conization and/or hysterectomy have been described by MARTIUS, TE LINDE, BALL, LYON et al., TOPEK, KAPLAN and KAUFMAN, and many others.

After arrival in the operating room the patient's urinary bladder is emptied by catheterization. (If hysterectomy is contemplated as the definitive procedure, a No. 14 or 16 Foley catheter is left indwelling.) The vagina is sponged dry. For many years operators have been scrubbing the vulva and vagina with soap and water prior to painting the cervix and vagina with Lugol's solution. It has been pointed out by numerous writers that the scrubbing and use of detergents should be discontinued.

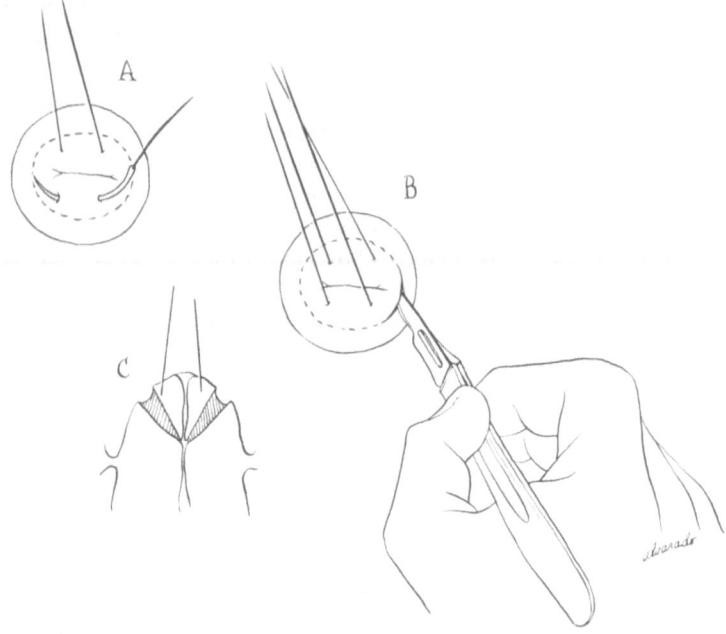

Fig. 1. A Traction sutures of braided silk are placed in the cervical area to be coned. B Incision is being made with No. 15 blade scalpel. C The conization specimen is being pulled away from the cervix. It should be conical, not cylindrical

At the present time we are of the opinion that 1% aqueous solution of toluidine blue dye applied to the cervix and vagina followed by destaining with 3% acetic acid as described by RICHART is more accurate than the Schiller test. One notes "the confluent areas of blue-staining epithelium adjacent to the squamocolumnar junction lying in the transformation zone". As a result, areas of nuclear concentration are thereby demonstrated. A figure of eight 0 chromic catgut suture is placed bilaterally at the cervicovaginal junction. When tied, these sutures serve for purposes of hemostasis and traction. Two sutures of braided silk are placed in the base of the cone to be removed as shown in Fig. 1 and as described by TWOMBLY at the last Clinical Meeting of the American Association of Obstetricians and Gynecologists.

Depending upon the results of the staining test a circular incision is made with a No. 15 scalpel blade. The mucous membrane peripheral to this incision is then freed for several millimeters. A cone of tissue is removed, care being taken to stay below the internal cervical os. The remaining portion of the cervical canal and the internal os are dilated and uterine curettage performed. Two or more figure of eight sutures may be required laterally to secure hemostasis.

Fig. 2 illustrates the overlapping of catgut sutures placed just below the cervico-vaginal junction as advocated by TOPEK et al. in pregnant patients. He points out that the tying of the sutures results in constriction of the cervix. They state: "As a result, the cervix is somewhat puckered and everted; therefore, the scalpel should be directed to obtain what appears to be a very shallow cone. However, the cone will be adequate and sufficiently deep. Further hemostasis and correction of the defect of the cervix can then be accomplished by figure of eight or Sturmdorf type sutures

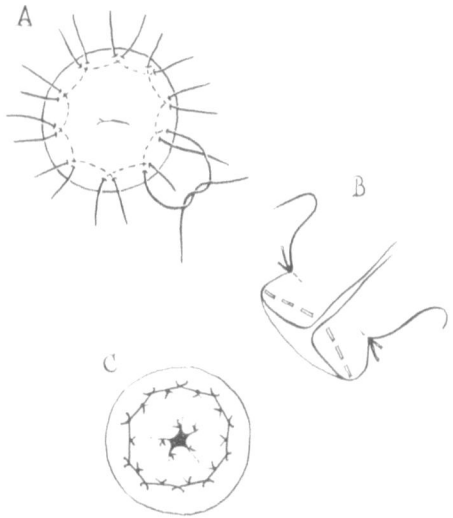

Fig. 2. A Overlapping 0 chromic catgut sutures in the cervix of pregnancy. B Lateral sutures have been tied. C Sturmdorf and Fig. 8 sutures are used for tissue approximation and for hemostasis

again employing atraumatic 0 chromic catgut. He also describes in considerable detail technic for hysterectomy with vaginal cuff, stating, "To date we have accomplished this procedure in 42 patients. 32 of them had epidermoid carcinoma in situ of the cervix".

Hysterectomy with Vaginal Cuff Excision

When definitive treatment for carcinoma in situ of the cervix is required, a hysterectomy with removal of approximately 2.5 cm of vaginal cuff is advisable. As pointed out by PARKER et al. vaginal hysterectomy has been performed in preference to abdominal hysterectomy in recent years for the reason that the necessary margin of vaginal cuff can be delineated under direct vision and the hysterectomy may be combined with colpoplastic repair when indicated. Furthermore, as LASH has stated, the extracervical lesions disclosed by the Schiller test can be excised. The use of braided silk traction sutures placed in the four quadrants at the cervicovaginal junction is advocated. The vaginal cuff is developed posteriorly beginning in the midline about 2.5 cm from the cervicovaginal junction. In extending the incision laterally one should follow a ruga. This also facilitates removing a satisfactory amount of tissue in all directions. Anteriorly the mucous membrane is freed by dissection from the bladder, laterally from the ligaments and posteriorly from the peritoneum

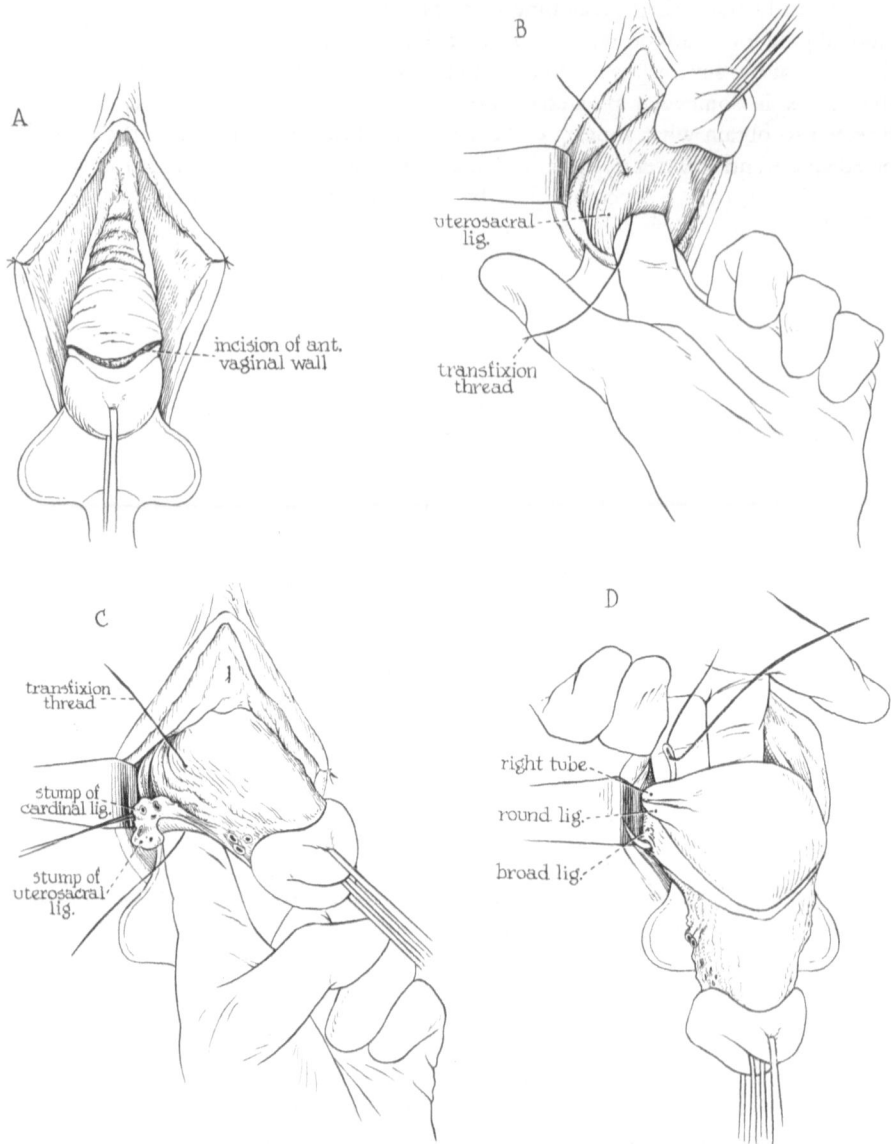

Fig. 3 A—E. Vaginal hysterectomy in a case having only a small area of carcinoma in situ of the cervix. A The incision is made anteriorly, after having been made posteriorly and bilaterally. B The right uterosacral ligament is being tied with 0 chromic catgut, which is the suture material to be used throughout the operation. C The uterosacral and cardinal ligaments have been ligated with transfixion sutures and a similar suture is being placed to ligate the uterine blood vessels. D The salpinx, the top of the broad ligament, and the round and utero-ovarian ligaments are being ligated. E The peritoneum of the cul-de-sac of Douglas is ready for closure. A pursestring suture will be used

of the cul-de-sac of Douglas. The cuff should be adequate to cover a 7.5 × 7.5 cm 12 ply gauze sponge. The cuff is sutured and the cul-de-sac of Douglas is entered. The supravaginal septum is cut and the vesicouterine fold of peritoneum opened. Hysterectomy is performed by modified Martius technic (see Fig. 3). The tubes and ovaries are inspected and palpated. In the absence of disease they are left in situ. If the patient has an enterocele it is corrected. If she has stress urinary incontinence a urethrocystopexy is done. If there is a rectocele and/or perineal relaxation repair is done. If the patient is a candidate for an abdominal rather than a vaginal hysterectomy we favor development of the cuff vaginally as described. We suture it over the previously mentioned sponge prior to placing the patient in the usual position for laparotomy. Upon opening the abdomen the tubes and ovaries are carefully inspected and palpated. Their removal will be predicated upon their condition and not on the age of the patient. If the appendix vermiformis is in view it will be removed prior to packing off the intestines; otherwise, its extirpation will be done subsequent to the hysterectomy and exploration of the peritoneal cavity.

Patients treated by hysterectomy and vaginal cuff excision should be followed at regular intervals by examination and cytologic studies to detect the occasional

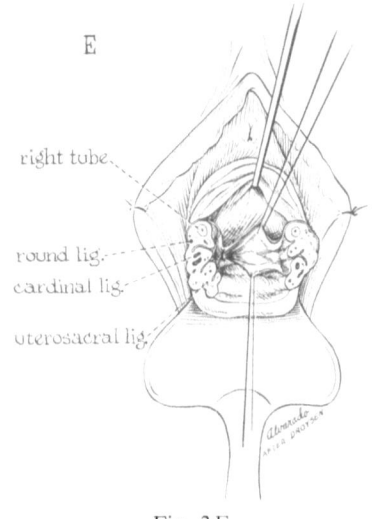

Fig. 3 E

recurrence of intraepithelial cancer or the development of an invasive lesion in the vagina.

Osoba, Cavanagh and Rutledge, Rutledge and Ibanez, and Malinak et al. have studied the conization-hysterectomy time interval. They concluded: "Hysterectomy should be postponed for at least 3 weeks and probably longer after conization, unless the conization specimen can be accurately studied immediately so that a definitive operation may be carried out without delay." In 1962 Kaufman et al. discussed "use of the refrigerated microtome for rapid diagnosis of cervical conization specimens". In this and subsequent articles they have demonstrated the accuracy of frozen section study and enumerated the advantage of the cryostat method. Among these is definitive surgery, including hysterectomy, which can be performed while the patient is still on the operating table. If she proves to have invasive carcinoma she can be treated definitively by the application of radium or by the indicated surgery. Immediate complications of conization such as bleeding and infection while the patient waits for the surgery are eliminated when the hysterectomy is promptly done.

The morbidity rate associated with the delay in performing hysterectomy following conization is markedly decreased; furthermore, the hospital stay is definitely shortened. At the Southern Baptist Hospital we have been impressed by the advantages of the cryostat technic. In cases of carcinoma in situ of the cervix requiring hysterectomy the cone has been obtained and hysterectomy done under the same anesthetic upon receipt of the pathologist's report. As Kaufman states: "The psychologic advantages for the patient when immediate hysterectomy is performed are quite obvious. The prospect of having to return to the operating room for a second operative procedure or having to delay surgery for 6 or more weeks, is not a pleasant one for most patients."

Carcinoma in Situ During Pregnancy

GREENE and PECKHAM have proved that physiologic gestational cervical epithelium does not mimic carcinoma in situ. MUSSEY and DECKER, WALTERS and REAGAN, and WRIGHT have written convincingly regarding the accuracy of cytologic diagnosis of cervical conditions during pregnancy. At the present time one might surmise that the incidence of cervical carcinoma in situ in pregnancy is about 1 in 333 gestations. The hazards of bleeding, infection, abortion, premature labor, and malfunction of the cervix during labor are discussed in articles on cervical carcinoma during pregnancy by many contributors.

Table 1. *Reported recurrence of carcinoma in situ of cervix uteri*

Author	Years	Pts.	Pts. treated	Recurr.
FRIEDELL et al.	1926—52	235	232	0
FENNELL	1927—53	118	106	3
GUSBERG and MARSHALL	1927—59	327	310	6
MUSSEY and SOULE	1932—47	842	838	5
PARKER et al.	1947—53	485	361	2
Cox	1955—59	146	146	3
DEVEREUX and EDWARDS	1960—64	632	630	6
		2785	2623	25

The number of pregnant patients included in the series of the authors listed in Table 1 are as follows: PARKER et al. 64, DEVEREUX and EDWARDS 19, MUSSEY and SOULE 14, Cox 7. In 1960 BEECHAM and ANDROS reported a series of 26 conization biopsies of the cervix during pregnancy. Indications, technics, and complications were discussed. In the same year FERGUSON and BROWN reported 50 cases. In 1964 BOUTSELIS and ULIERY discussed 69 cases of intraepithelial carcinoma of the cervix in pregnancy. The incidence of complications following diagnostic conization was 14.5%. They stated: "Definitive therapy for carcinoma in situ at our institution consists of total hysterectomy, resection of 1 to 2 cm of upper vaginal cuff and preservation of the ovaries during the childbearing years." WILLIAMS and TURNBULL reported on 76 cases, 52 of whom were treated by modified Wertheim hysterectomy, 10 had conizations of the cervix alone. In 1966 MOORE et al. discuss the diagnosis and management of 42 cases with carcinoma in situ of the cervix during pregnancy. They included "not only cancer confined to the surface epithelium and/or the endocervical glands but also microscopic stromal invasion — i.e. that limited to the outer 2 to 3 mm of subepithelial tissue". 29 patients were subjected to cervical conization and this was the definitive treatment in 25% of the patients. At the time of the report they had not observed any recurrences after definitive treatment (conization or hysterectomy). Four cesarean hysterectomies were performed.

In a review of 60 cases of pregnancy following the conservative treatment of 50 patients with cervical carcinoma in situ GREEN stated: "Whilst the number of patients with abortion, premature labour, or cervical dystocia was not greatly increased it is considered that cervical conization tends to cause these complications and should be replaced by a ring-type biopsy when future childbearing is important."

FESTE et al. reported 13 cesarean section hysterectomies with abnormal cervico-vaginal smears detected late in pregnancy. They stated: "Cervical conization with cryostat frozen section evaluation followed by immediate cesarean section hysterectomy was carried out on 9 patients. 4 patients had cesarean section hysterectomy performed at term because of a prior conization during pregnancy revealing squamous cell carcinoma in situ." Among their conclusions we find: "Cesarean section hysterectomy with removal of 2 to 3 cm of vaginal cuff is advocated at or near term as treatment for those patients diagnosed as having squamous cell carcinoma in situ of the cervix during pregnancy when no further childbearing is desired. When more children are desired, vaginal delivery is allowed."

MUSSEY and DECKER gave a case analysis of 95 patients who were pregnant either when intraepithelial carcinoma was proved or within the previous year. Of the 37 patients having intraepithelial carcinoma during pregnancy gestation was interrupted in 12 instances by hysterectomy. Four additional patients had carcinoma in situ in association with incomplete abortion and the remaining 21 women were allowed to complete their pregnancies after the malignancy had been proved. Their final comment is: "Cancer of the cervix in association with pregnancy need no longer be a tragic situation, difficult to manage, if adequate cytologic screening of the cervix of the young women becomes an integral part of the practice of every physician managing prenatal care. Conization, although not as extensive as in the nonpregnant patient, can and should include adequate tissue for examination by means of the frozen section technic, permitting prompt and accurate evaluation by the pathologist as to the inclusion of a margin of normal epithelium and the exclusion of microinvasion. Iodine staining of the cervix prior to conization also helps delineate the size of the cone. We conclude that cauterization should be used for hemostasis after conization since there is a much lower incidence of residual intraepithelial carcinoma in cervices thus treated."

At the 1967 meeting of the Pacific Coast Obstetrical and Gynecological Society, JONES et al. reported the results of 5 years of cytodetection of the cervix during pregnancy in the Prenatal Clinics of the City and County of Los Angeles, stating: "Patients with carcinoma in situ, regardless of age, were urged to have a hysterectomy. Women desirous of having children and willing to continue cytologic examinations every 3 months, were treated by the diagnostic conization. Only half of these patients have honored their commitment to appear regularly for cytologic follow-up".

Carcinoma in Situ at Charity Hospital at New Orleans

Table 2 bearing the caption Charity Hospital of Louisiana at New Orleans concerns an institution of over 2400 beds which are divided in two Medical School Services called Units.

TORRES states that on the Louisiana State University Unit of Charity Hospital at New Orleans the number of carcinoma in situ of the cervix cases were as follows: 1960 — 33, 1961 — 23, 1962 — 32, 1963 — 51, 1964 — 50, 1965 — 71, 1966 — 42, 1967 — 25. He stated: "As you may know, in 1963 we extended our cytology screening program in our clinics and the increased number of cases diagnosed from 1963 through 1965 I believe is a reflection of the efficacy of this program. The drop that has occurred in 1966 and 1967 I believe is due to the fact that we are reaching a prevalence figure in our static clinic population which is approaching the figure for new case incidence per year." The total number of cases diagnosed during pregnancy for the years 1956 through 1966 was 34. In an article published in 1964 TORRES et al.

Table 2. *Charity Hospital of Louisiana at New Orleans*

	1963	1964	1965	1966	1967	Total
Births	8983	8785	8925	8741	8444	43878
Cesareans	439	382	333	315	312	1781
C. Hysterectomies	100	94	86	92	77	449
Gyn. Admits.	2471	2467	2669	2603	2298	12508
Abd. Hysterectomies	469	543	311	401	317	2041
Vag. Hysterectomies	451	332	774	620	408	2585

Table 3. *Charity Hospital of Louisiana at New Orleans. Tulane unit*

	1963	1964	1965	1966	1967	Total
Births	4432	4361	4481	4345	4244	21863
Cesareans	131	118	124	150	137	660
C. Hysterectomies	44	54	49	49	63	259
Gyn. Admits.	1236	1209	1250	1066	1127	5888
Abd. Hysterectomies	143	148	145	151	215	802
Vag. Hysterectomies	265	275	298	285	216	1339

Table 4. *Cervical carcinoma in situ at New Orleans Charity Hospital. Tulane unit*

	1960	1961	1962	1963	1964	1965	Total
Cases	14	39	22	21	31	15	142
White/nonwhite	2/12	7/32	2/20	7/14	9/22	0/15	27/115
Conization only	1[a]	2	1[a]	0	1	1	6
Wide cuff hysterectomy	10	28	17	17	23	11	106
Abd. hysterectomy	2	5	2	2	3	3	17
Vag. hysterectomy	1	2	0	1	2	0	6
Cesarean hysterectomy	0	1	0	0	1	1	3
Residual tumor in hyst. specimen	0	0	0	9	12	7	28

[a] Pregnant.

stated: "It is possible that dysplasia may precede the appearance of carcinoma in situ. For this reason it is necessary to follow patients with dysplasia carefully, since an unknown number of these women may develop carcinoma".

Table 3 provides some data concerning the Tulane University Unit at Charity Hospital. During the last 5 years for which records were available 142 proved cases of cervical carcinoma in situ were tabulated. See Table 4. Of these 27 were white and 115 nonwhite. The oldest patient was 82 and the youngest 15. As shown, wide cuff hysterectomy was the most often employed type of treatment. Most of these were done by the vaginal route. The 17 patients who had abdominal hysterectomy without wide cuff excision included such emergency cases as ruptured tubo-ovarian abscesses and ectopic pregnancies. A number of the hysterectomies were for myomas. There were 3 cesarean hysterectomies. Residual tumor was found in 28 hysterectomy specimens. In 1963 a patient who had a recurrence after wide cuff vaginal hysterectomy was given the benefit of exenteration. She is alive today.

Carcinoma in Situ at Southern Baptist Hospital

The Southern Baptist Hospital is a private institution of approximately 475 beds. In contrast to Charity Hospital where the patient population is overwhelmingly non-white the patients at this institution are white. Table 5 shows that there were 21,008

Table 5. *Southern Baptist Hospital, New Orleans*

	1963	1964	1965	1966	1967	Total
Births	4426	4417	4121	4106	3938	21008
Cesareans	283	238	228	224	183	1156
C. hysterectomies	32	26	42	46	33	179
Gyn. admits.	1888	1707	1776	1859	1852	9082
Abd. hysterectomies	353	514	576	613	652	2708
Vag. hysterectomies	343	342	364	365	319	1733

Table 6. *Southern Baptist Hospital. Carcinoma in situ of cervix uteri*

	1963	1964	1965	1966	1967	Total
Patients	9	12	19	25	22	87
Conization only	1	2	3	4	4	14
Conization and hysterectomy	1	4	6	7	5	23
Conization, hysterectomy later	5	5	6	7	11	34
Abdominal hysterectomy	7	7	10	7	13	44
Vaginal hysterectomy	0	2	5	11	5	23
Excision cervical stump	0	0	0	1	0	1
Cesarean hysterectomy	1	0	0	1	0	2
Residual tumor in hyst. specimen	4	8	5	10	8	35

1966 1 case radio-therapy.
1964 and 1965 1 case D and C and cervical biopsy.

births there during the past 5 years. This exceeds the number of white births at Charity Hospital during the same time. Records of 87 patients having cervical carcinoma in situ from January 1, 1963 through 1967 were available for perusal. Treatment of 73 patients was by 27 obstetricians-gynecologists. 5 patients were treated by general surgeons, the same number by general practitioners, and 3 were operated upon by Residents in Obstetrics and Gynecology. 1 patient deserted after histologic diagnosis had been made but before hysterectomy with wide cuff excision could be performed.

In Table 6 it will be noticed that 23 patients were given the benefit of hysterectomy as soon as the pathologist reported on examination of the conization specimen by the cryostat method. As previously stated, this is a time and money-saving procedure. Even more important, it prevents complications and dangers inherent in a second stage procedure, also anxiety. Two of the patients had cesarean hysterectomy. 35 hysterectomy specimens showed residual tumor. During the last few years more of the operators have been employing the wide cuff hysterectomy technic. Fig. 4 shows the age distribution of the patients. The youngest patient was 20 and the oldest was 65. HAJDU et al. reported the case of a 15 year old Negress who had two babies. He mentioned the 16 year old patient of FERGUSON.

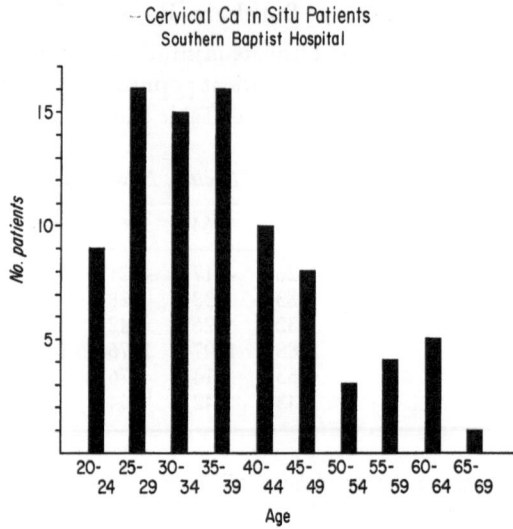

Fig. 4. Most of the patients in the Southern Baptist Hospital series were in the 25 through 39 years age groups

References

ADELMAN, H. C., and S. J. HAJDU: Amer. J. Obstet. Gynec. 98, 173—179 (1967).
ANDERSON, S. G., and E. B. LINTON: Amer. J. Obstet. Gynec. 98, 113—116 (1967).
ASHLEY, D. J. B.: J. Obstet. Gynaec. Brit. Cwlth 73, 382—389 (1966).
— J. Obstet. Gynaec. Brit. Cwlth 73, 372—381 (1966).
BALL, T. W.: Gynecologic surgery and urology, 2nd. ed. St. Louis, Mo.: C. V. Mosby Co. 1963.
BEECHAM, C. T., and G. J. ANDROS: Obstet. and Gynec. 16, 521—526 (1960).
BOUTSELIS, J. G., and J. C. ULLERY: Amer. J. Obstet. Gynec. 90, 593—609 (1964).
CAVANAGH, D., and F. RUTLEDGE: Amer. J. Obstet. Gynec. 80, 53—59 (1960).
Cox, B. S.: J. Obstet. Gynaec. Brit. Cwlth 74, 723—727 (1967).
CRISP, W. E., H. SHALAUTA, and W. A. BENNETT: Obstet. and Gynec. 31, 755—758 (1968).
CROSSEN, H. S., and R. J. CROSSEN: Operative gynecology, 6th ed. St. Louis, Mo.: C. V. Mosby Co. 1948.
CULLEN, T. S.: Cancer of the uterus. New York: Appleton 1900
DEMIN, V. N.: Obstet. and Gynec. 31, 288—292 (1968).
DEVEREUX, W. P., and C. L. EDWARDS: Amer. J. Obstet. Gynec. 98, 497—508 (1967).
DOUGLAS, R. G., GEORGE N. PAPANICOLAOU: Trans. Amer. gynec. Soc. 85, 185—187 (1962).
FENNELL, R. H., JR.: Cancer (Philad.) 9, 374—384 (1956).
FERGUSON, J. H., and G. C. BROWN: Surg. Gynec. Obstet. 111, 603—606 (1960).
FESTE, J. R., R. H. KAUFMAN, H. L. SKOGLAND, and N. H. TOPEK: Amer. J. Obstet. Gynec. 95, 763—768 (1966).
FRIEDELL, G. H., A. T. HERTIG, and P. A. YOUNGE: Carcinoma in situ of uterine cervix: A study of 235 cases from the Free Hospital for Women. Springfield: Thomas 1960.
FUNNELL, J. D., and J. A. MERRILL: Surg. Gynec. Obstet. 117, 15—19 (1963).

GREEN, G. H.: Amer. J. Obstet. Gynec. **94**, 1009—1022 (1966).
— Obstet. Gynaec. Brit. Cwlth **73**, 897—902 (1966).
— Int. Surg. **47**, 511—517 (1967).
GREENE, R. R., and B. B. PECKHAM: Amer. J. Obstet. Gynec. **75**, 551—564 (1948).
GUSBERG, S. G., and D. MARSHALL: Obstet. and Gynec. **19**, 713—720 (1962).
HAJDU, S. I., J. SO-BOSITA, and A. B. LITTLE: Amer. J. Obstet. Gynec. **100**, 1154—1155 (1968).
HALLGRIMISSON, J. T.: Acta obstet. gynec. scand. **46**, 268—272 (1967).
HAMPERL, H.: (1) Med. Welt (Stuttg.) **20**, 1098—1100 (1965).
— (2) Geburtsh. u. Frauenheilk. **25/2**, 105—111 (1965).
HESTER, L. L., and R. A. READ: Amer. J. Obstet. Gynec. **80**, 715—721 (1960).
HINSELMANN, H.: Zbl. Gynäk. **51**, 901—903 (1927).
JONES, E. G., C. P. SCHWINN, W. K. BULLOCK, A. VARGA, J. E. DUNN, H. FRIEDMAN JR., and J. WEIR: Amer. J. Obstet. Gynec. **101**, 298—306 (1968).
JONES, H. W., JR., K. P. KATAYAMA, A. STAFL, and H. J. DAVIS: Obstet. and Gynec. **30**, 790—805 (1967).
KAPLAN, A. L., and R. H. KAUFMAN: Clin. Obstet. Gynec. **10**, 871—878 (1967).
KAUFMAN, R. H.: Clin. Obstet. Gynec. **10**, 838—852 (1967).
—, J. T. ABBOTT, and W. C. SCHEIHING: Amer. J. Obstet. Gynec. **84**, 107—112 (1962).
—, O. G. JANES, and H. A. COX: Amer. J. Obstet. Gynec. **92**, 71—77 (1965).
—, W. A. JOHNSON, J. J. SPJUT, and A. SMITH: Acta cytol. (Philad.) **11**, 272—278 (1967).
KOTTMEIER, H. L.: Official classification of certain pelvic malignancies approved. A.C.O.G. Newsletter, p. 11—12, Feb. 1963.
LASH, A. F.: Int. Surg. **47**, 518—527 (1967).
LAUCHLAN, S. C., and D. W. PENNER: Cancer (Philad.) **20**, 2250—2254 (1967).
LYON, J. B., S. HAJJAR, and J. D. THOMPSON: Sth. med. J. (Bgham, Ala.) **58**, 937—944 (1965).
MALINAK, L. R., R. A. JEFFREY JR., and W. J. DUNN: Obstet. and Gynec. **23**, 317—329 (1964).
MARCUS, S. L.: Amer. J. Obstet. Gynec. **80**, 802—812 (1960).
MARTIUS, H.: Martius' gynecological operations, 7th. ed. Translation by McCALL, M. L., and K. A. BOLTEN. Boston: Little, Brown & Co. 1956.
McCANN, S. W., A. MICKAL, and J. T. CRAPANZANO: Personal communication.
MEYER, R.: Zbl. Gynäk. **47**, 946—960 (1923).
MOORE, J. G., R. G. WELLS, and D. G. MORTON: Obstet. and Gynec. **27**, 307—318 (1966).
MUSSEY, E., and D. G. DECKER: Amer. J. Obstet. Gynec. **97**, 30—38 (1967).
—, and E. H. SOULE: Amer. J. Obstet. Gynec. **77**, 957—972 (1959).
NEWMAN, W., and J. K. CROMER: Surg. Gynec. Obstet. **108**, 273—281 (1959).
OSOBA, D.: Canad. med. Ass. J. **79**, 805—809 (1958).
PAPANICOLAOU, G. N.: Proc. Third Race Betterment Conference, 1928.
—, and H. F. TRAUT: Diagnosis of uterine cancer by the vaginal smear. Cambridge: Commonwealth Fund, Harvard Univ. Press 1943.
PARKER, R. T., W. K. CUYLER, L. A. KAUFMAN, B. CARTER, W. L. THOMAS, R. N. CREADICK, V. H. TURNER, C. H. PEETE JR., and W. B. CHERNEY: Amer. J. Obstet. Gynec. **80**, 693—710 (1960).
PEMBERTON, F. A., and G. V. S. SMITH: Amer. J. Obstet. Gynec. **17**, 165—176 (1929).
RICHART, R. M.: Amer. J. Obstet. Gynec. **86**, 703—712 (1963).
ROGERS, R. S., and J. H. WILLIAMS: Amer. J. Obstet. Gynec. **98**, 488—494 (1967).
RUBIN, I.: Amer. J. Obstet. Gynec. **62**, 668—676 (1910).
RUTLEDGE, R., and M. L. IBANEZ: Amer. J. Obstet. Gynec. **83**, 1208—1213 (1961).
SCHIFFER, M. A., J. J. GREENE, W. POMERANCE, and A. MOLTZ: Amer. J. Obstet. Gynec. **93**, 889—895 (1965).
SCHILLER, W.: Surg. Gynec. Obstet. **56**, 210—222 (1933).
SCHAUENSTEIN, W.: Arch. Gynäk. **85**, 576—616 (1908).
SCHOTTLANDER, J., and F. KERMAUNER: Zur Kenntnis des Uteruskarzinoms. Berlin: Karger 1912.
SILBAR, E. L., and J. D. WOODRUFF: Obstet. and Gynec. **27**, 89—97 (1966).
STAHMANN, F. S.: S. Dak. J. Med. Pharm. **17**, 19—21 (1964).

TE LINDE, R. W.: Operative gynecology, 3rd. ed. Philadelphia (Pa.): J. B. Lippincott Co. 1962.
—, G. A. GLAVIN, and H. W. JONES JR.: Amer. J. Obstet. Gynec. **74**, 792—803 (1957).
TORRES, J. E.: Personal communication.
— Acta cytol. (Philad.) **8**, 284—287 (1964).
TOPEK, N. H.: Clin. Obstet. Gynec. **10**, 853—870 (1967).
TWOMBLY, G. H.: Personal communication.
WALTERS, W. D., and J. W. REAGAN: Amer. J. clin. Path. **26**, 1314—1325 (1956).
WILLIAMS, T. J., and K. E. TURNBULL: Obstet. and Gynec. **24**, 857—864 (1964).
WRIGHT, L.: J. Obstet. Gynaec. Brit. Cwlth **68**, 771—777 (1961).
YOUNGE, P. A., A. T. HERTIG, and D. ARMSTRONG: Amer. J. Obstet. Gynec. **58**, 867—895 (1949).

Tendencies of Growth and Spread of Squamous Cell Cancer of the Cervix

K. G. OBER

HENRIKSEN (1960) one time compared the spread of carcinoma of the cervix with a roulette. While the ball is rolling, nobody knows where it is going to stop. The probability, however, which will promise success to repeated putting in, may be small or great. Therefore the stakes are limited.

In selecting an operation for cancer most surgeons are considering different point of views. Among them are evaluation of the disease and its potential spread in the individual case.

We evaluated specimens of 379[1] abdominal operations for squamous cell carcinomas using identical techniques. The *continuous* growth of the primary tumor we use to catch by histologic giant sections of the cervix in two directions (MATUSCHKA, 1962; OBER and HUHN, 1962) in different blocks and between 100 and 300 micron in thickness (Figs. 1, 2, 4). For evaluating the *discontinuous* growth, which in most of the cases is lymph node involvement, during operation the lymph nodes are fixed in different containers with alcoholic Bouin's fluid. After a careful count the lymph nodes also are worked up by step sections (HUHN, 1964; OBER and HUHN, 1962; VOGT-HOERNER and GÉRARD-MARCHANT, 1958). In individual operations between 9 and 54 lymph nodes were removed, in the average 20.7. Altogether 7845 nodes were examined.

Extensive abdominal surgery for cancer with lymphadenectomy we carry out for those tumors almost exclusively which already can be seen with the naked eyes or palpated with the fingers. Figs. 1a—c show typically those squamous cell carcinomas which I want to talk about. Adenocarcinomas, cancers of the mesonephric duct, mucoepidermoids, mixed tumors — that are neoplasms which represent approximately 5 to 6% of all cervical cancers — are left out. Ignored are also carcinomas of the vagina (Fig. 1d) which at occasion unfoundedly may have been called cervical

---

[1] Part of these observations had been reported by the author together with HUHN in 1962 from the University-Women-Hospital in Cologne. Professor Dr. C. KAUFMANN was kind enough to place at our disposal another 110 specimens, which were obtained by the same surgical technique since 1962.

cancers. Quite frequently we operate the large, extensive tumors of the cervix where we still can find a dissection plane against the pelvic wall (Figs. 1 b and c).

Fairly scarce among our specimens are the small, clinically easily detectable carcinomas (Fig. 1 a). They can be operated well. Therefore these cases are probably treated more often outside of the large hospitals. Our material contains a relatively

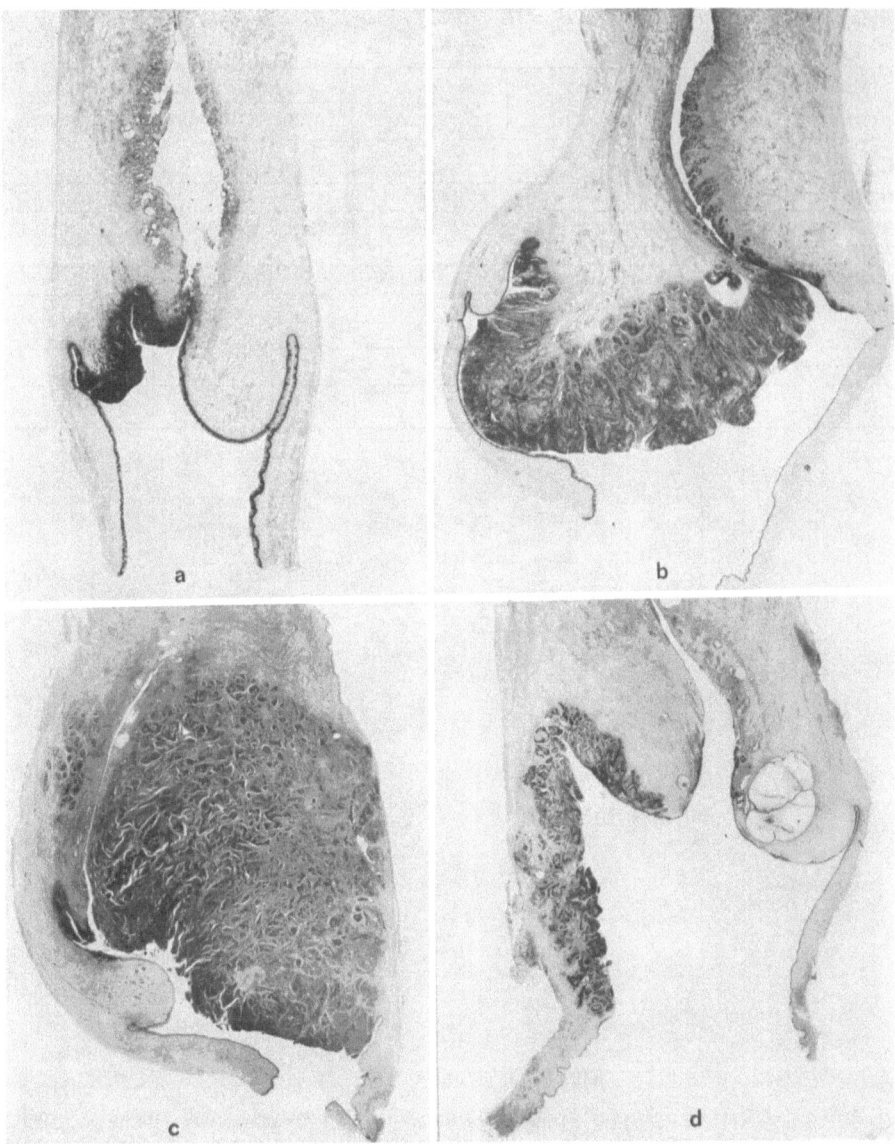

Fig. 1. Three different forms of typical carcinomas (a, b, c) compared with a high-located carcinoma of the vagina (d). b and c represent typically exophytic and endophytic growth. The carcinoma in situ which can be seen in d just above the cervical glands does not justify a classification as cervical carcinoma. The major portion of the cornified squamous cell carcinoma most likely has derived from the upper part of the vagina

575

small group of early cancers (Table 1)[2]. We also did not evaluate specimens of women who had received irradiation treatment prior to surgery or of others who required some type of evisceration procedure after a previous operation or curative radiation treatment had failed.

Furthermore our cases are selected from another point of view: I consider the fact that one can avoid castration to be one of the great advantages of the surgical

Table 1. *Relation of continuous growth of the primary tumor to involvement of lymph nodes of pelvic wall*

Continuous growth of the primary tumor	Cases	Lymph node involvement	
		Tumor cell emboli	Metastases
Microcarcinomata	25	—	—
Strictly confined to the cervix	207	12	35
Laterally still within the cervix, but involvement of the vagina	24	1	13
Involvement of the boundary zone(s)	70	3	24
Involvement of the boundary zone(s) and the vagina	19	—	10
Involvement of the paratissues	34	2	21
Total	379	18	103

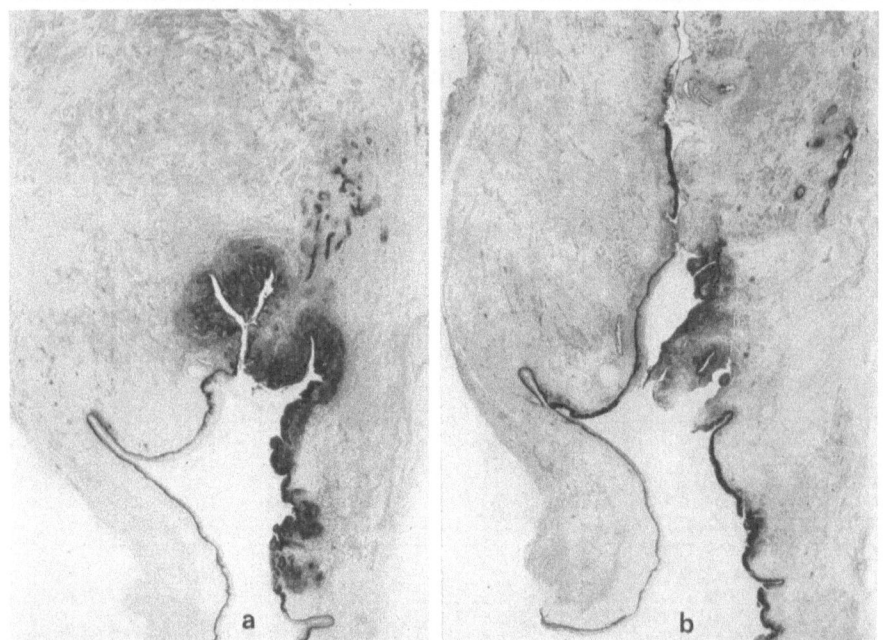

Fig. 2. Step sections of a surgical specimen disclose that a relatively small cancer — which indeed is extending to the upper fifth of the vagina — continuously makes a breach towards the paratissues. The boundary zone of the cervix has not been crossed yet. There is no case in our material showing this type of spread into the paracervical tissues

[2] 21 of the so-called microcarcinomata are coming from the hospital in Cologne. The special problems of this group were brought to attention by KAUFMANN, OBER and HUHN on hand of 130 observations in 1965.

approach. Therefore in Erlangen we almost never use irradiation treatment following surgery. Quite independent of the surgical risk we predominantly operate on women under 50 years of age — even in relatively advanced carcinomas.

Since beginning of this century one was concerned with the problem of growth and spread of carcinoma of the cervix. Until about 10 years ago the investigations of BRUNET (1905), KUNDRAT (1903) and SCHEIB (1909) carried great weight. Even today they are the fundament of the international classification of stages. It is certain that cervical cancers have the special feature of remaining within the pelvis for a relatively long period of time. But the assumption that rather seldom tumors are reaching the paracervical, the paravaginal and occasionally even the parametrial tissue by continuous growth — without leading to metastases to the regional lymph nodes — today is not valid any more.

The definition of the *continuous* growth is obvious: The most advanced proliferations of the tumor still will have to be in cellular connection with the primary growth (Figs. 2a and b). The term *discontinuous* spread we apply for metastases (HAMPERL, 1960). The latter don't have direct contact with the primary tumor anymore (Figs. 3b and c, as well as Figs. 4b and c).

In regard to the *continuous* spread of cervical cancers the following suggestion appears necessary: There does not exist a distinct boundary line between the cervix and the paracervical tissues, which in the beginning of this century caused investigators to register a transgression of the cervix by the tumor for 1 or 2 mm. Cervix and paracervical tissues cannot be separated accurately from each other. A *boundary zone* (Fig. 4a) up to 5 mm in depth is located in between (OBER and HUHN, 1962; OBER and MEINRENKEN, 1964). Not before this zone has been exceeded by the cancer one is allowed to call it a *continuous* spread into the paracervical tissues. The surgeon is not able to recognize this boundary zone during the operation. A simple hysterectomy will always take place within this zone. Only operations which take along a portion of the paravaginal and paracervical tissues, will include the boundary zone too.

The diagnosis of metastases to the lymph nodes may be a problem. One will have to reckon with entirely different interpretations. A metastasis exists in that case only when a conglomerate of tumor cells has become firmly adherent to the lymph node (Figs. 3c, 5c; HAMPERL, 1960; HUHN, 1967). Not unusually seen are pictures of cell complexes which are found to be free within the marginal sinus (Figs. 3a, partly 3b). These should not be called metastases. This term should be used even less for the rather varying pictures of epithelial complexes, which at times assume more solid, more frequently, however, glandular forms. These so-called "gland inclusions", which HUHN had observed in 1962 in more than 40% of all women who had radical abdominal surgery because of a cervical cancer were partly interpreted as cancer metastases early this century.

Tables 1 and 2 show a classification of the 379 observations in regard to the *continuous* as well as the *discontinuous* spread. Most of our observations are referring to tumors which histologically clearly were limited to the cervix (207 of 379). $1/_6$ of them (35 of 207) showed metastases of the lymph nodes. $1/_4$ of the cancers (89 of 379) had proliferated continuously up to the boundary zone. A good $1/_3$ of those showed involvement of lymph nodes (34 of 89). About $1/_{10}$ (34 of 379) of the surgical specimens showed the *continuous* penetration of the boundary zone into the paravaginal, paracervical and parauterine tissues. 21 of these 34 cases showed *discontinuous* involvement of the lymph nodes.

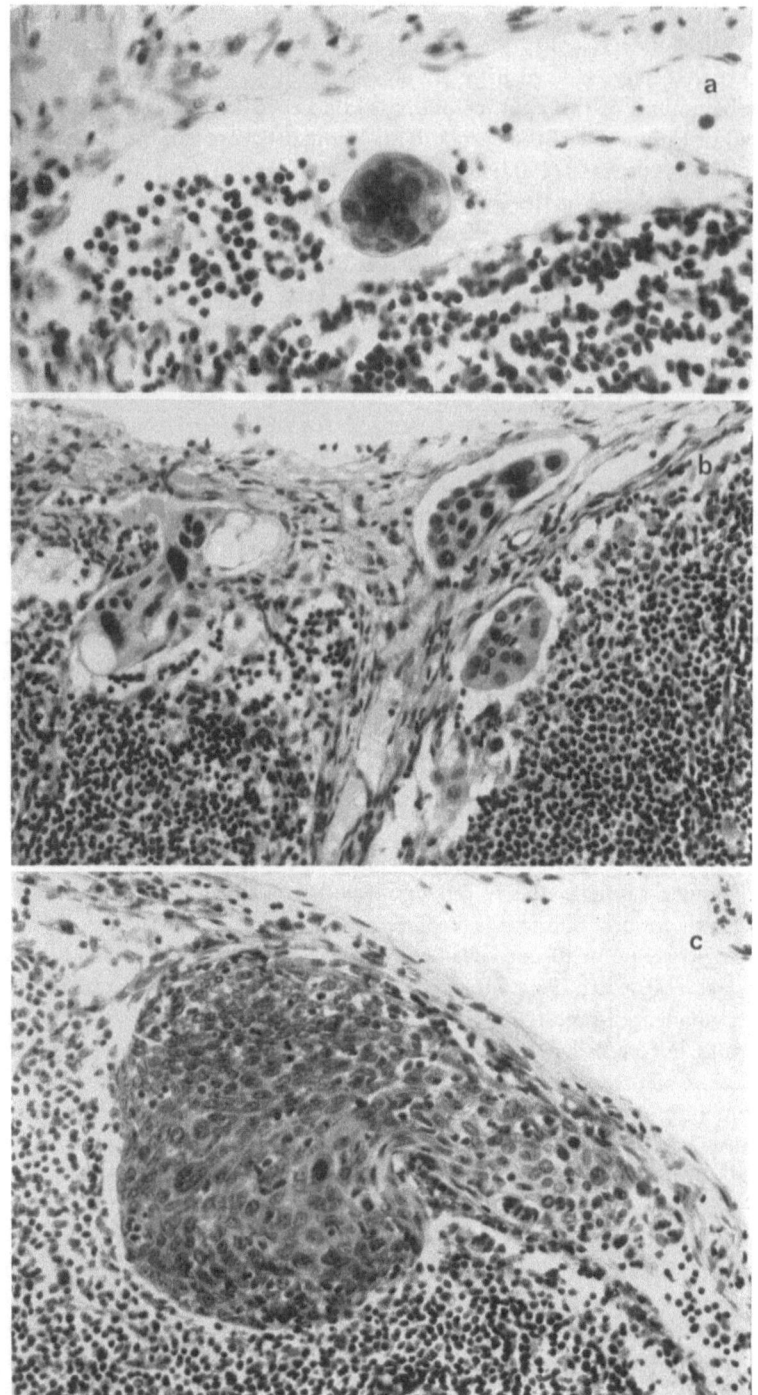

Fig. 3a—c. Sections of marginal zones of different lymph nodes. a Tumor cell embolism within a marginal sinus. b To the left and above there is a very small metastasis partly showing vacuolar degeneration. To the right there are two tumor cell emboli, which cannot be interpreted as metastases for certain from this section. c Small metastasis

It happens extremely seldom that small cancers having the size of a lentil or a pea already have metastasized. The metastasis of the smallest carcinoma which we discovered with our technique is shown in Fig. 5. The probability of metastatic spread of these carcinomas may be in the range of 1:50 up to 1:100. These estimations are supported, however, by additional 112 observations of women with microcarcinomata, which were not treated with lymphadenectomy (compare with page 582).

The quantitative correlation between size of tumor and involvement of lymph nodes was secured by HUHN in 1964 through careful measurements.

Table 1 points out to an observation which at first surprised us very much. Tumors which have not reached the boundary zone, but which have expanded with an infiltrative growing pattern towards the vagina — which frequently occurs beneath the vaginal epithelium — show metastases of the lymph nodes in approximately half of the cases (13 of 24). The same relationship exists in tumors which have

Table 2. *The relation of continuous growth of the primary tumor to its discontinuous spread to the paratissues*

Continuous growth of the primary tumor	Cases	Involvement of paratissues by discontinuous spread
Microcarcinomata	25	—
Strictly confined to the cervix	207	14 (+ 1 TE)[a]
Laterally still within the cervix, but involvement of the vagina	24	2 (+ 2 TE)
Involvement of the boundary zone(s)	70	11 (+ 1 TE)
Involvement of the boundary zone(s) and the vagina	19	4
Involvement of the paratissues	34	4
Total	379	35 (+ 4 TE)

[a] TE = tumor cell emboli only.

proliferated into the boundary zone and at the same time into the vagina (10 of 19). Our numbers are small. One will have to watch this problem in the future more carefully. A short remark regarding the stage grouping appears important at this point. Stage IIa usually can be diagnosed easily. Many patients of our entire patient collective would have been grouped stage II b or even stage III by other colleagues. With this point in mind our observation in regard to the involvement of the vagina appears to be important.

Table 2 shows a survey of the correlation of the *continuous* spread to the *discontinuous* metastazising into the parametria. Tables 3 and 4 points out that with ignoring the involvement of the boundary zone two thirds (46 of 64) of the women with involvement of the parametria had metastases to the lymph nodes of the pelvic wall. For considerations in respect to surgical techniques this appears to be important.

One could discuss the question, whether involvement of the parametrial lymph nodes better ought to be added to involvement of the nodes of the pelvic wall. From the pathologic-anatomical point of view it would appear reasonable to include

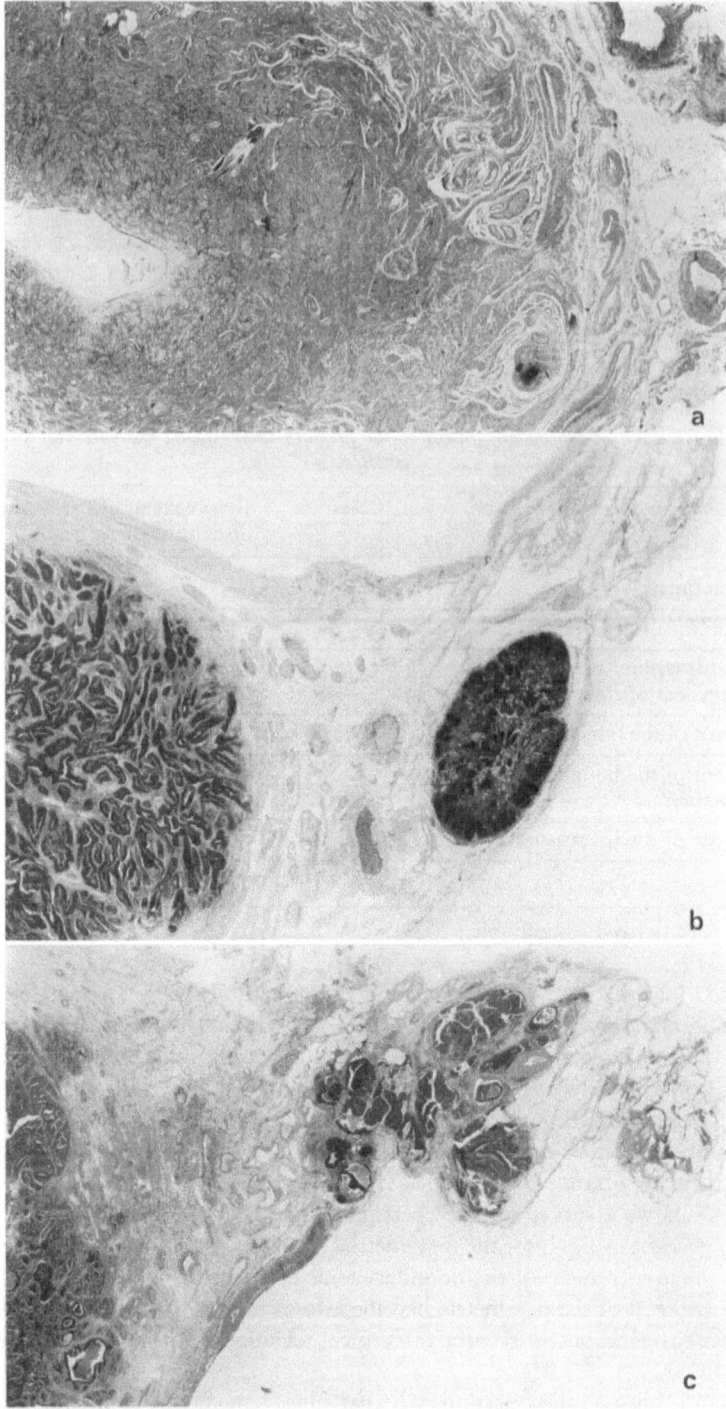

Fig. 4. (Legends see page 581)

Table 3. *Coincidence of discontinuous involvement of the paratissues and the lymph nodes of pelvic wall*

Continuous growth of the primary tumor	Paratissues			Lymph nodes	
	Strictly confined to lymph node(s)		TE[a]	TE[a]	Metastases
Strictly confined to the cervix	9	5	1	—	13
Laterally still within the cervix, but infiltration of the vagina	1	1	2	—	3
Involvement of the lateral boundary zone(s)	7	4	1	1	6
Involvement of the lateral boundary zone(s) and the vagina	1	3	—	—	3
Involvement of the paratissues	1	3	—	1	3
Total	19	16	4	2	28

[a] TE = tumor cell emboli only.

Table 4. *Coincidence of cancer involvement of the paratissues (contin. a./or discontin.) and lymph nodes of pelvic wall*

Continuous growth of the primary tumor	Paratissues	Lymph nodes
Strictly confined to the cervix	14 (+ 1 TE)[a]	13
Laterally still within the cervix, but infiltration of the vagina	2 (+ 2 TE)	3
Involvement of the lateral boundary zone(s)	11 (+ 1 TE)	6 (+ 1 TE)
Involvement of the lateral boundary zone(s) and the vagina	4	3
Involvement of the paratissues	33	21 (+ 2 TE)
Total	64 (+ 4 TE)	46 (+ 3 TE)

[a] TE = tumor cell emboli only.

lymph nodes of the paratissues to those of the pelvic wall. However, surgeons usually should class them as belonging to the paratissues since the deciding difference between vaginal and abdominal operations is the fact that the vaginal approach will not permit removal of lymph nodes of the pelvic wall while lymph nodes of the paratissues can be taken along. One may also ask, whether once in a while the *discontinuous* involvement of the parametrial tissues may have happened retrogradely. The latter we were not able to prove for certain in operable cases. Sometimes metastases in the parametrial tissues will develop apparently in spite of progressively more dilating vessels (Fig. 4c).

Fig. 4. a Boundary zone between cervix and paracervical tissues. One cannot draw an exact boundary line between cervix and supporting tissues. There is a vascular boundary zone, which may be up to 5 mm in depth in the non-magnified specimen. b A lymph node in the paracervical tissues filled out with cancer in a tumor which did not yet invade the boundary zone for certain. c A metastasis in the paracervical tissues which developed by discontinuous growth obviously without relation to lymph nodes. This metastasis has derived from a tumor which had invaded the boundary zone

In regard to the side localization of the continuous and discontinuous spread of cancer our material did not reveal any significant differences (Table 5). The preference of one side does not appear to play a role, neither in continuous growth nor in development of metastases. The relationship of left to right is in *unilateral* spread with involvement of the boundary zone 43:34, with penetration of the boundary zone 11:9, with the *discontinuous* involvement of parametrium 15:15 and with the involvement of the lymph nodes of the pelvic wall 31:37.

It does not make any difference whether the tumors are extending to both sides or to one side only: The involvement of the lymph nodes of the pelvic wall shows approximately twice as frequently metastazising to the lymph nodes around the common iliac vessels and to lymph nodes of the so-called vessel triangle between the external and internal iliac vessels than to the lymph nodes of the paravesical and pararectal area. Involvement of the inguinal lymph nodes we did not yet observe in operable cases.

Table 5. *Localization of unilateral continuous and discontinuous spread of cancer*

	Continuous spread		Discontinuous spread	
	Left	Right	Left	Right
Boundary zone	43	34		
Paratissues	11	9	15	15
Lymph nodes of pelvic wall			31	37

Usually we don't resect the hypogastric vein together with its branches. The 3 or 4 gluteal lymph nodes therefore are not removed. I cannot tell much about their involvement, but I want to stress this point: Among 148 women who were observed at least for 3 years and who did not have metastases of the lymph nodes when examined with our method, there were four women until now who showed a recurrence in the pelvis.

There appear to be physicians who carry out the vaginal cancer operation taking along the paravaginal, paracervical and parametrial tissues assuming that very small cancers are able to make a breach by growing continuously into the paratissues without involving the lymph nodes of the pelvic wall (Fig. 6). We did never see this type of picture although we have removed in healthy tissues additional 112 microcarcinomas by simple hysterectomy or conization beside the 25 microcancers mentioned in Table 1. We have observed these cases now for at least 3* years (KAUFMANN et al., 1965; OBER, 1965). So it has to be very rare. Figs. 2a and b demonstrate this type of expansion in an extreme manner *within* the cervix and without involving the boundary zone and the paracervical tissues. This type of infiltration is a very rare one. Only 3% of the tumors are growing this way; more than 90% have a shallow front of invasion (OBER and HUHN, 1962). The typical manner a cervical cancer encroaches is shown by the Figs. 4b and c. The *discontinuous* spread within the paracervical or paravaginal tissues (Figs. 4b and c) very often goes along with involving lymph nodes of the pelvic wall (28 of 34 cases; Table 3).

To the question regarding metastazising into the ovaries we can contribute just a little, as we don't castrate most of our patients — no matter how big the primary tumor may be. None of these women later on did run a course indicating that we had

---

* 4 years in May 1969.

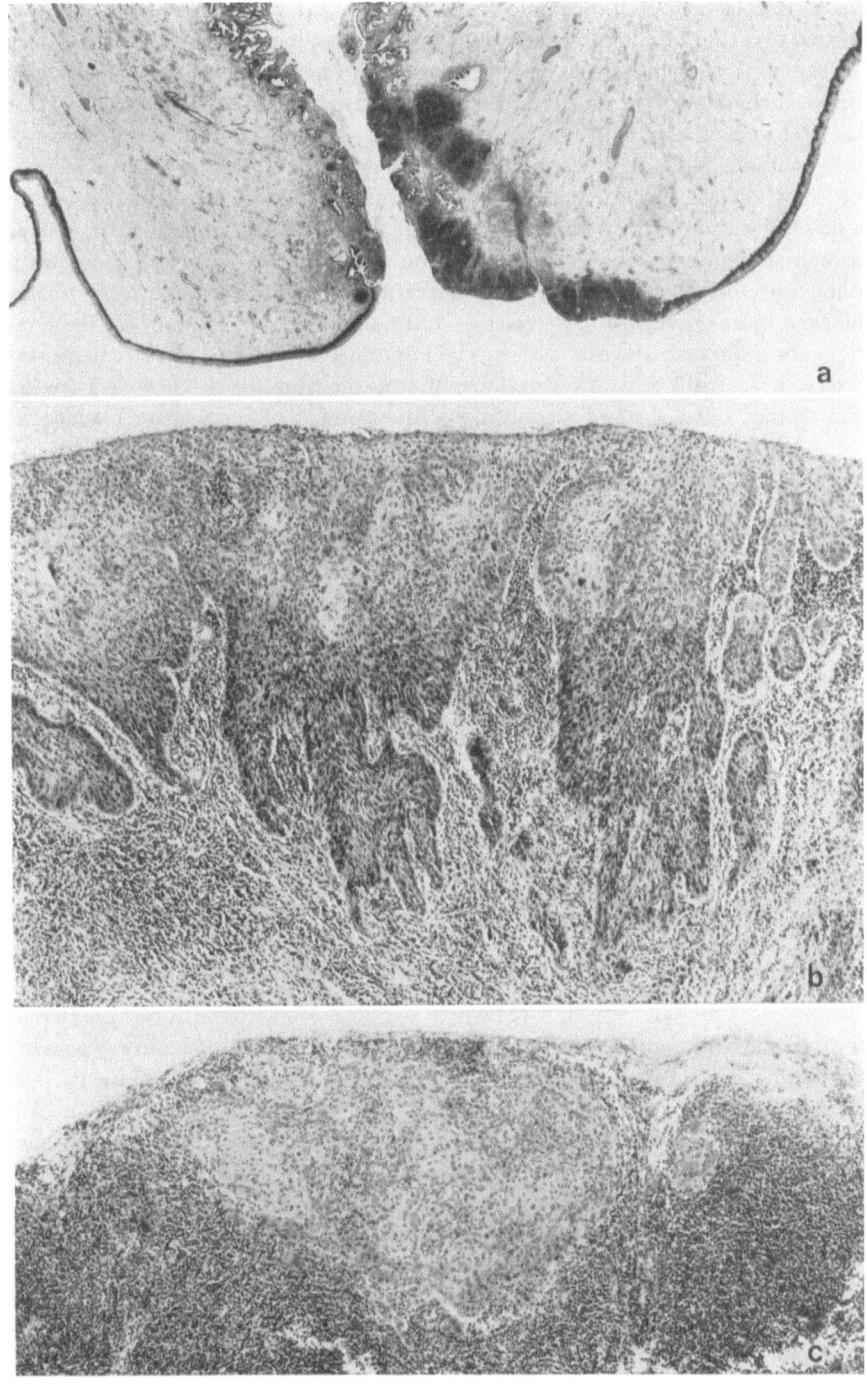

Fig. 5. a Pocket-lens magnification of the smallest cancer we observed with metastases to the lymph nodes of the pelvic wall. b Low magnification of the border section of this tumor. c Low magnification of the metastasis within a lymph node of the pelvic wall

left a metastasis behind. Twice only we had to deal with patients, which could not be operated grossly radical and who had already ovarian metastases.

Very important appears to be another question which has been a matter of discussion lately (FRIEDELL and PARSONS, 1961; HENRIKSEN, 1960; OBER and HUHN, 1962; PARSONS et al., 1959; PARSONS et al., 1960): What is the significance of cancers which infiltrate the bladder continuously or invade the rectum as a consequence of preexisting disease (for instance peritonitis within the pelvis or endometriosis in the cul-de-sac) without already having penetrated the paracervical, paravaginal and parametrial tissues by continuous expansion up to the pelvic wall? Here we are dealing with those cases which one could treat operatively without trying irradiation. One even must operate in these cases — ultraradically! I am looking for these conditions for more than 10 years with special interest. I never saw a primary invasion of the rectum with still present surgical line of cleavage from the pelvic wall. I saw only seven women, who showed a continuous involvement of the urinary bladder who

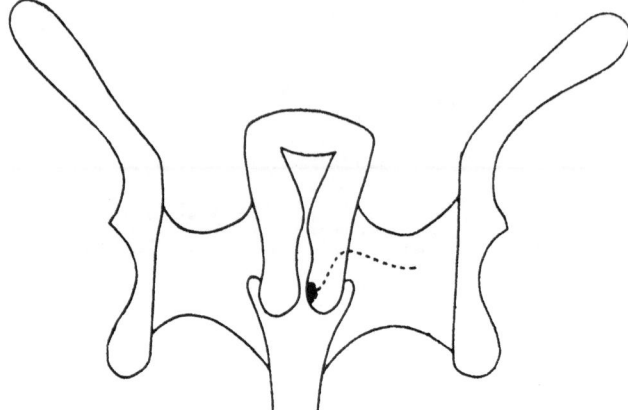

Fig. 6. The idea of the continuous manner of expansion of a very small carcinoma of the cervix which that physician should have in mind who would use in this case the vaginal operation described by SCHUCHARDT-SCHAUTA-AMREICH. (After OBER, 1965)

still presented a dissection plane to the pelvic wall. In regard to the involvement of the rectum I could imagine that high-located vaginal cancers may cause misinterpretations (Fig. 1 d).

As a gynecologist, who is doing the surgery and who uses to evaluate the specimens histologically himself, I should emphazise therapeutic points of view, of course.

Cervical cancers, which an experienced gynecologist can recognize clinically, always should be operated in conjunction with lymphadenectomy. The metastatic spread to lymph nodes of the pelvic wall plays a much greater role than one thought in earlier times. If a simple hysterectomy is not be sufficient, one will have to remove the paravaginal and paracervical tissues and the lymph nodes of the pelvic wall as well. If one considers an involvement of the paratissues, consequently one will have to lymphadenectomize.

In very small cancers (microcarcinomata) one does not have to consider a spread into the paravaginal, paracervical or parametrial tissues. The probability of metastazising into the lymph nodes is extremely small. In cases of great surgical risk or those cases of increased risk to irradiation this knowledge will facilitate the choice of treatment.

Provided one should not find any metastases of lymph nodes following extensive surgery and most thorough examination of the specimens, the probability of a so-called "recurrence" is extremely small. This knowledge may at times be of great help for answering the question of castration during an operation or for making the decision of irradiation treatment following an operation.

References

BRUNET, G.: Z. Geburtsh. Gynäk. **56**, 1 (1905).
FRIEDELL, G. H., and J. B. GRAHAM: Surg. Gynec. Obstet. **108**, 513 (1959).
—, and L. PARSONS: Cancer (Philad.) **14**, 42 (1961).
HAMPERL, H.: Langenbecks Arch. klin. Chir. **295**, 22 (1960).
HENRIKSEN, E.: Amer. J. Obstet. Gynec. **80**, 1919 (1960).
HUHN, F. O.: Geburtsh. u. Frauenheilk. **22**, 335 (1962).
— Virchows Arch. path. Anat. **325**, 84 (1962).
— Die Lymphknotenveränderungen beim Cervixcarcinom und die Beziehungen Tumorgröße und lymphogene Ausbreitung. Habil.-Schrift, Köln 1964.
— Morphologie der Tumormetastasierung, Krebsforschung und Krebsbekämpfung, VI, p. 238 (1967).
KAUFMANN, C., K. G. OBER und F. O. HUHN: Geburtsh. u. Frauenheilk. **25**, 112 (1965).
KUNDRAT, R.: Arch. Gynäk. **69**, 355 (1903).
MATUSCHKA, M.: Geburtsh. u. Frauenheilk. **22**, 497 (1962).
OBER, K. G.: Geburtsh. u. Frauenheilk. **25**, 464 (1965).
—, u. F. O. HUHN: Arch. Gynäk. **197**, 262 (1962).
—, u. H. MEINRENKEN: Gynäkologische Operationen. In: GULEKE u. ZENKER, Allgemeine und spezielle chirurgische Operationslehre, Band IX. Berlin-Göttingen-Heidelberg-New York: Springer 1964.
PARSONS, L., F. CESARE, and G. H. FRIEDELL: Surg. Gynec. Obstet. **109**, 279 (1959).
— — — Ann. Surg. **151**, 961 (1960).
SCHEIB, A.: Arch. Gynäk. **87**, 241 (1909).
VOGT-HOERNER, G., et R. GERARD-MARCHANT: Bull. Cancer **45**, 446 (1958).

Individualization of Treatment for Cancer of the Cervix*

S. B. GUSBERG, and JOHN RUDOLPH

If one is to take the position that we should individualize treatment for cancer of the cervix as we do for other diseases according to the patient's age, general health and outlook one must choose between the two excellent modalities of treatment available to us: radical surgery and radiotherapy, or elect combinations thereof. In order to make this choice dependent upon patient factors rather than therapist factors, by which I mean the training, temperament, departmental policy or other variables related to the physician in charge, we must utilize the biological parameters clinically available for this decision.

If we assume that all other factors are equal, we might start with the premise that radiation will give as good a cure rate in Stage I or Stage II ("the operable stages") as will radical surgery, with a lesser rate of therapeutic mortality and a greater rate of

* From The Department of Obstetrics and Gynecology of The Mount Sinai School of Medicine and Hospital. — This work was supported in part by The American Cancer Society: Grant No. T-7F. and by the U.S.P.H.S.

Table 1. *Mean survival rate in cancer of the cervix*[a]

Modality		No. of patients	5year survival rate
Stage I	Radiation	7,133	72.0%
	Combined	4,621	78.2%
	Surgery	391	71.8%
	Selected surgery	2,052	74.0%
Stage II	Radiation	12,120	53.8%
	Combined	6,407	55.7%
	Surgery	601	52.5%
	Selected surgery	2,523	50.6%

[a] From 14th Annual Report, Stockholm.

Table 2. *Radiation therapy — selected*

Stage I with 80% + survival:

Institution	% 5year survival	No. of patients
Erlangen, Germany	80.4	97
Munich I, Germany	83.8	290
Munich II, Germany	93.8	64
Warsaw, Poland	80.7	378
Stockholm, Sweden	86.4	471
Houston, USA	86.6	216
San Francisco, USA	83.9	143
Leningrad, USSR	82.6	161
Mean 84.8		1,820/7,133

% of total number subjected to Rx in clinics with this high cure rate = 25.5%. Rx = treatment

Table 3. *Radiation therapy — selected*

Stage II with 60% + survival:

Institution	% 5year survival	No. of patients
Innsbruck, Austria	70.6	126
Brno, Czechoslovakia	67.0	91
Brno II, Czechoslovakia	67.8	118
Aarhus, Denmark	65.1	338
Erlangen, Germany	66.1	230
Munich I, Germany	69.9	1,002
Munich II, Germany	66.3	187
Tubingen, Germany	63.5	348
Wurzburg, Germany	67.5	114
Rotterdam, Netherlands	64.4	149
Stockholm, Sweden	60.0	1,094
Houston, USA	69.9	382
Mean 66.5		4,179/12,120

% of total number subjected to Rx in clinics with this high cure rate were = 34.4%.

applicability. However, we must acknowledge that "all other factors" are not equal and that experience with the management and follow-up of these patients forces one to the conclusion that some patients will benefit more from surgical treatment in an era when the morbidity from such surgery is small and early, whereas the morbidity from radiotherapeutic treatment may be commulative and late, when the life expectancy of the "cured" young patient (and we see more of these with early lesions) may be 30 to 40 years, when there are simple observations to be made that suggest that the requirement of radiation for a particular tumor of low sensitivity will be of such an intensity as to increase the tissue damage over that usually seen under skilled treatment. This message of individualization will not influence those wedded to a technical rather than a biological concept of cancer treatment.

To make a comparison between the survival rates following surgery and irradiation treatments in Stages I and II carcinoma of the cervix we have analyzed the tabulations in the 14th Annual Report compiled in Stockholm in an effort to seek out data

Table 4. *Combined treatment — selected*

Stage I with 80% + survival:

Institution	% 5year survival	No. of patients
Frankfurt, Germany	80.8	271
Kiel, Germany	88.0	133
Wuppertal, Germany	82.1	240
Kumamoto, Japan	83.8	111
Okayama, Japan	85.6	299
Tokyo, Japan	85.0	333
Bucharest, Rumania	81.3	252
Zurich, Switzerland	88.0	125
Moscow, USSR	90.6	159
Ljubljana, Yogoslavia	84.2	330
Zagreb, Yugoslavia	80.8	266
Mean 84.6		2,519/4,621

% of total number of patients subjected to Rx in clinics with this high cure rate = 54.5%.

that could influence our choice of treatment. One quickly finds that there is little difference in the "cure" rate of surgery or irradiation in either the average group or those selected for superiority of reported result (Tables 1 to 7).

The criteria used for the selection of clinics and the definition of treatment groups are outlined below:

1. Each clinic must have had at least 100 patients in Stage I and Stage II or a combined total of at least 200 patients (1956 to 1960).

2. *Radiation:* The majority of the patients (greater than 70%) with Stage I and II lesions must have received primary radiotherapy.

3. *Surgery:* The majority of the patients (greater than 50%) in Stages I and II must have had primary surgery.

4. *Combined:* The majority of the patients (greater than 50%) in Stages I and II received surgery and planned pre or postoperative radiotherapy.

5. *Selected surgery:* A group wherein more than 30%, but less than 50%, of Stage I and II lesions received primary surgery. The remainder received radiotherapy.

Table 5. *Combined treatment — selected*

Stage II with 60% + survival:

Institution	% 5year survival	No. of patients
Vienna, Austria	61.5	122
Frankfurt, Germany	64.9	245
Okayama, Japan	68.4	820
Tokyo, Japan	69.9	530
Amsterdam, Netherlands	62.2	193
Zurich, Switzerland	63.8	130
Zagreb, Yugoslavia	62.2	429
Mean 64.7		2,469/6,407

% of total number of patients subjected to Rx in clinics with this high cure rate = 38.3%.

Table 6. *Surgical treatment in selected clinics*

Stage I with survival rate 80% +:

Institution	% 5year survival	No. of patients
Nagasaki, Japan	86.0	50
Heidelberg, Germany	80.4	184
Boston, USA	80.3	132
Col.-Presby., N.Y., USA	80.6	139
Mean 81.3		505/2,443

% of total number of patients subjected to Rx in clinics with this high cure rate = 20.6%.

Stage II with survival rate 60% +:

Institution	% 5year survival	No. of patients
Nagasaki, Japan	70.1	137
Paris, Inst. G-Roussy	61.9	202
Mean 66.0		339/3,124

% of total number of patients subjected to Rx in clinics with this high cure rate = 10.8%.

Table 7. *Selected superior survival rates*

	Stage I survival	% applicable	Stage II survival	% applicable
Radiation	84.8	25.5	66.5	34.4
Combined	84.6	54.5	64.7	38.3
Surgery	81.3	20.6	66.0	10.8

Selection of clinics reporting 80% + survival in Stage I and 60% + in Stage II.

It is noteworthy that the clinics reporting a combined treatment of planned radio-therapy and surgery, showed some superiority both in survival rate and the percentage of patients to whom the superior treatment was being offered, but it is difficult to assay the role of selection in these figures.

Furthermore when the rate of major injury from each modality was inspected in the literature, there was little to choose between radiotherapy and surgery, though here once more the combined treatment seemed to show a higher rate. One must quickly add that the rates of injury shown here (Tables 8 to 12) are high for modern

Table 8. *Criteria for major injury in Rx of carcinoma of cervix*

Surgery	Radiation
Fistula	Fistula
Rectal	Rectal
Ureteral	Ureteral
Vesical	Vesical
Intestinal obstruction stricture	Stricture
Ureteral	Ureteral
	Rectal
Thromboembolic hemorrhage	Persistent proctitis and cystitis

Table 9. *A comparison of % injuries in relation to mode of treatment*

Mode	% injury
Surgery	13.1
Combined	16.9
Radiation	11.6

Table 10. *Surgical injury in operable carcinoma of the cervix*

Senior author	% injury
CALAME	13.0
BRUNSCHWIG	22.4
MASTERSON	5.0
MEIGS	11.0
YAGI	2.1
SYMMONDS	4.0
GREEN	20.3
LOUROS	2.8
GRAHAM	17.0
Mean 13.1	

Table 11. *Combined treatment in carcinoma of the cervix*

Senior author	% injury
TALBERT	15.0
HURTEAU	16.9
CRAWFORD	13.0
STALLWORTHY	0.0
GREISS	22.2
GRAHAM	34.0
Mean 16.9	

Table 12. *Radiation injury in carcinoma of the cervix*

Senior author	% injury
KOTTMEIER	3.9
SHERMAN	17.0
HURTEAU	7.5
CRAWFORD	20.0
GRAHAM	6.0
CALAME	16.3
GREISS	9.1
Mean 11.6	

treatment and they are declining for all modalities, as greater therapeutic precision and more careful selection of mode has prevailed.

If then, we cannot depend upon survival rate or injury rate for the selection of treatment in an operable patient with carcinoma of the cervix in those clinics where treatment by either mode is available we must turn to a more careful analysis of the patient and her tumor for help in this decision; we have chosen a radiosensitivity test based on a test dose technique.

Radiosensitivity and the Test Dose Technique

Three factors concerned with the cure of tumors by radiation are: (1) Excellence of treatment, (2) Radiation sensitivity and (3) Virulence of the tumor. As Gynecologists perhaps we are not privileged to discuss publicly the excellence of any radiotherapeutic treatment. However, I shall briefly refer to our study of these other factors as they influence our choice of treatment.

We have described before our Test Dose Technique with the administration of a provocative quantity of radiation, small enough so that it does not interfere with later surgical treatment or the precise planning of the geometry of radiotherapeutic treatment yet large enough to produce a spectrum of response. We have used in the past several experimental approaches to this test, including 3,000 R (250 KV, 15ma, 43 cm target-skin distance, half value layer 2 mm Cu) in 500 R daily exposures, via transvaginal cone, or 800 r × 2, 24 h apart, or external irradiation of 1,600 rads by supervoltage (Cobalt 60 or Betatron) but we have now standardized our test by giving 400 Rads × 3 in 3 days with external irradiation via parallel opposing fields (Betatron, whole pelvis technique) and continuation of treatment to 2000 Rads while awaiting the proper interval for the response biopsies. Control biopsies are taken in quadrants in healthy sectors of tumors and repeated on the 11th day after the onset of the test dose, i.e. 1 week after the test dose is concluded. The continuation of irradiation in the interval permits continuity of treatment if radiotherapeutic treatment is elected; this interval of 1 week may be used in addition for the general work-up required of patients with cervix cancer.

Tissue sections and tissue smears are made from these biopsies and stained by the previously described techniques for histologic, cytomorphologic and cytochemical reactions and, in addition, fixed in osmic acid for electron microscopic study.

There are three types of tumor cell reaction indicating responsiveness to irradiation: 1. death and dissolution of cells; 2. increased differentiation of cells; 3. radiocytologic reactions indicating the probability of irreversible cell injury such as (a) enlargement of cells and cell nuclei, (b) enlargement of nucleoli (RNA) and (c) alteration in chromatin material (DNA) with an apparent early increase followed by relative decline. As you know our testing studies are based in general upon the sensitivity of the reproductive apparatus of the cell to injury by irradiation while the organelles, more directly or more secondarily related to protein synthesis, seem to carry on with less sensitivity to the time of virtual explosion or dissolution of the cell.

The method is relatively simple and reproduceable and can be used in any laboratory where there is a pathologist available who will study radiation change in cells and tissues. We have used more elaborate quantitative methods but at present they are still too laborious for clinical application.

Response and Result

The incidence of good response in our series is close to 70%, in this analysis 68.1% without significant variation from stage to stage.

You have perhaps been accustomed to the philosophy that tumors that shrink early recur early, in this way prohibiting early prognosis of healing under radiation. We do not find this to be true. Indeed you will note that the initial response of these tumors to the test dose, i.e. 1 week following the administration of this relatively small amount of irradiation, enabled us to make a reasonably good estimate of the final response. In this group of patients, for example, where the radiotherapeutic mode was chosen without respect to the outcome of radiosensitivity testing, you will note that the relative cure rate in Stage I and II (excluding small Stage I's — Stage I-b and microcarcinomas — Stage I-a) was 72.1% whereas the relative cure rate for those with poor radiosensitivity testing declined to 32.5%; those of Stage II extent appeared to show the widest disparity. That the factors of radiosensitivity and virulence are intertwined may be seen from the following table wherein we have shown the result attained by the clinical use of radiosensitivity testing. In this group patients of Stage I and II extent with poor radiosensitivity testing were subjected to radical hysterectomy and we were able to bring the relative cure rate to 56% (Table 13).

Table 13. *CA cervix — Stages I and II. Response and treatment*

	No.	Cure
RST good-radiation	123	72.1%
RST poor-radiation	47	32.5%[a]
RST poor-surgery	28	56.0%[a]

[a] Significant at .05 level.

This appears to be a significantly better result for these individuals than that to be expected with continuation of radiotherapy but not as good as that for those with a good radiosensitivity testing response treated in the radiotherapeutic group above described.

As a relatively modest approach to the problem of virulence by the use of a parameter readily available to clinical study before treatment we investigated the presence or absence of lymphatic invasion in the control biopsy. This proved to be a valuable index for in the "good" radiosensitivity testing group we found an 86% relative cure rate in those without lymphatic invasion, but a 39.4% cure rate only in those with good radiosensitivity testing with positive lymphatic invasion. Expressed in another way those with good response who were living and well showed a 14.9% incidence of lymphatic invasion in the control biopsies, whereas those who recurred showed a 72.8% incidence (almost five times greater). This virulence factor has not been applied clinically as yet, but it could persuade us to use combinations of surgery and radiotherapy for this group. We have some small, statistically insignificant evidence that the lymphatic invasion factor did not effect the outcome in those patients treated surgically as much as it did those treated radiotherapeutically, which we shall pursue.

Discussion

It may be that we can raise our cure rate by this radiosensitivity testing program but our purpose may be more properly expressed as an effort to find the parameters that will enable us to choose between two relatively good forms of treatment or combinations thereof most suited to the needs of the individual patient. It is clear that most of the factors in tumor healing, like those of tumor growth, are as yet unknown. At the same time I believe we have wasted much time and energy in polemic displays suggesting that our modalities of treatment are competitive rather than complementary. We should get on with further biological studies now possible by more sophisticated techniques to assay the response to radiation and the areas where surgery may be more efficiently utilized with the premise that tumors of greater resistence or higher virulence may require an intensity of radiotherapy that makes the cost in normal tissue damage prohibitive and we may then alter our radiation approach or substitute surgery or combine it with surgery, in a manner that will most suit the nature of the tumor and its host.

References

Annual Report Vol. 14 — Stockholm. Ed. HANS L. KOTTMEIER.
BRUNSCHWIG, A., and H. R. K. BARBER: Obstet. and Gynec. 27, 21—29 (1966).
CALAME, R., and R. WALLACH: Surg. Gynec. Obstet. 125, 39—44 (1967).
CRAWFORD, E., L. S. ROBINSON, and J. VAUGHT: Amer. J. Obstet. Gynec. 91, 480—485 (1965).
GRAHAM, J., R. GRAHAM, and M. SCHULZ: Amer. J. Obstet. Gynec. 89, 421—431 (1964).
GREEN, T. H.: Progress in the management and prevention of the urologic complications of radical Wertheim hysterectomy. In: MEIGS, J. V., and S. H. STURGIS, Ed., Progress in gynecology, p. 646—659. New York: Grune and Stratton, Publishers 1963.
—, J. V. MEIGS, H. ULFELDER, and R. CURTIN: Obstet. and Gynec. 20, 293—312 (1962).
GREISS, F. C.: Combined radiation and surgical treatment for carcinoma of the uterine cervix. In: LEWIS, G. C., W. B. WENTZ, and R. M. JAFFE, Ed., New concepts in gynecological oncology, p. 133—141. F. A. Davis Co., Publishers 1966.
—, D. D. BLAKE, and F. R. LOCK: Obstet. and Gynec. 18, 417—427 (1961).
GUSBERG, S. B.: Amer. J. Obstet. Gynec. 72, 804 (1956).
—, and G. G. HERMAN: Amer. J. Obstet. Gynec. 100, 627 (1968).
— — Amer. J. Obstet. Gynec. 87, 60 (1962).
HURTEAU, G. D., J. MORRIS, and C. H. CHANG: Amer. J. Obstet. Gynec. 95, 696—705 (1966).
KOTTMEIER, H. L.: Amer. J. Obstet. Gynec. 88, 854—866 (1964).
LIU, W., and J. V. MEIGS: Amer. J. Obstet. Gynec. 69, 1—32 (1955).
LOUROS, N. C.: Amer. J. Obstet. Gynec. 89, 432—438 (1964).
MASTERSON, J.: Clin. Obstet. Gynec. 10, 927—939 (1968).
SHERMAN, A. I., and H. M. CAMEL: Amer. J. Obstet. Gynec. 89, 439—452 (1964).
STALLWORTHY, J.: J. Amer. med. Ass. 195, 465—470 (1966).
SYMMONDS, R. E.: Amer. J. Obstet. Gynec. 94, 663—678 (1966).
TALBERT, L. M., L. PALUMBO, H. SHINGLETON, C. A. BREAM, and J. A. McGEE: Sth. med. J. (Bgham, Ala.) 58, 11—17 (1965).
YAGI, H.: Amer. J. Obstet. Gynec. 69, 32—47 (1955).

Abdominal Operations for Cervical Cancer

LANGDON PARSONS

Nearly 30 years after the resurgence of abdominal surgery for cervical cancer in the United States it is appropriate to review the experience and attempt to delineate the role it should play as the sole definitive mode of therapy.

Modern surgery makes it possible for us to adapt our therapy to the individual needs of the patient. We are aware of the fact that cancer of the cervix may be treated by either radiation or surgery. For Stages I and II we speak of having a choice in our selection of therapy. The choice does exist but only if there is equal competence in both fields.

A large portion of radiation therapy for cancer of the cervix is given by radiologists whose primary interest and training is in diagnosis rather than therapy. Similarly a great deal of surgery is performed by men who have limited knowledge of the life history of cervical cancer or the problems that they may encounter.

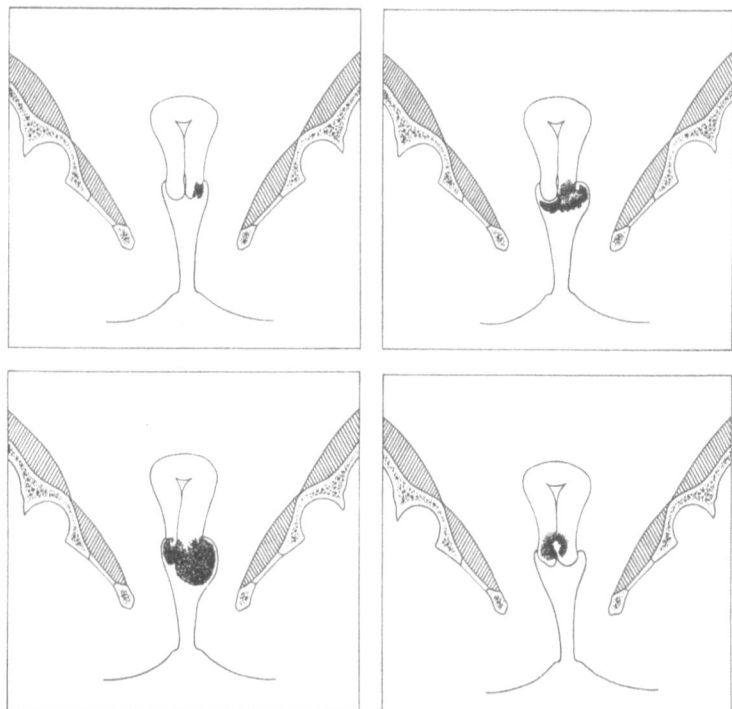

Fig. 1. Stage I cancer of the cervix. The lesion is confined to the cervix. It may be ulcerating or exfoliating

Unfortunately, despite the fact that radiation has improved and surgery has become more extensive, we still are not doing as well as we should for invasive cancer of the cervix. The most recent statistics, recounting the world experience as published in the 14th volume of the Annual Report on the results of treatment in carcinoma of the uterus and vagina, suggest that approximately 50% of all women with cervical cancer fail to survive the 5 year period.

It is my firm belief that cancer of the cervix is basically a local disease. We should be able to cure more patients than we do. It is possible to do so provided the therapy is well conceived and vigorously carried out.

The problem is not whether radiation or surgery will offer the highest percentage of cure in all cases seen but what is best for the individual. Within the scope of individualization abdominal surgery has a logical place in the management of cervical cancer.

The primary aim of surgery is to encompass all the tumor at the primary site and the areas to which it may be expected to extend, including the regional nodal areas. The indications for the abdominal surgical approach would seem to be well defined, but in the United States at least they appear to be much misunderstood and are variously interpreted. A considerable amount of confusion still exists as to (1) when to offer the patient surgery, (2) what the limitations of surgery are, and (3) how extensive the operation should be to be considered adequate.

In my opinion there would be less uncertainty of the role abdominal surgery should play if we had a better understanding of what it is that we are trying to accomplish. To have such understanding we must have a workable knowledge of the life history of the tumor we are dealing with. It has been well documented that the growth pattern of cervical cancer tends to confine it to the primary site and the immediate paracervical and paravaginal areas, with only a moderate degree of involvement of the regional nodes.

To be effective the operation chosen must have sufficient scope to encompass all the disease the patient may have. It is not reasonable to expect one standard operation will accomplish this in all patients and for all stages of the disease. The surgeon should have at his command and be familiar with the techniques of a number of different procedures so that he can tailor his operation to the amount of the patient's disease. It is no longer justifiable to force the patient to accept the only procedure the surgeon knows how to do.

There are two abdominal surgical procedures that may be employed. (1) The Wertheim Meigs' type of radical hysterectomy combined with pelvic lymphadenectomy. (2) The pelvic exenteration operations. The Wertheim operation is done as the sole definitive treatment in Stages I and II cervical cancer. The exenteration operations are primarily performed on patient who have failed to respond to adequate radiation therapy. There is, however, a place for the exenteration as primary definitive therapy. We are all aware that the clinical evaluation of the amount of disease present, since it is done with the examining finger alone, may be in error as much as 20%. In most instances this is on the side of more, rather than less, disease. The surgeon then should be prepared to remove the bladder or rectum and occasionally both, if he finds that he has underestimated the amount of disease and there is actually more cancer present than he anticipated. The only other alternative available to the surgeon is to discontinue the operation, mark the gross extent of the tumor with dura clips so that the radiologist has some idea of the amount and location of the disease and submit the patient to radiation therapy. It is not in the best interest of the patient to persist in continuing with a Wertheim procedure that is doomed to failure from the beginning.

This is one of the reasons why I prefer the abdominal rather than the vaginal surgical approach in cervical cancer. The radical Schauta Amreich procedure does not permit the flexibility present in the Wertheim Meigs' hysterectomy when the patients found to have more disease than was originally anticipated.

How well does the Wertheim Meigs' hysterectomy with pelvic node dissection meet the requirements of encompassing all of the cancer at the primary site and in the areas to which it may logically spread? It is my impression that in my own country too much of the surgery that is performed as definitive therapy is less than adequate. I believe this is so for two reasons. (1) The Wertheim type of hysterectomy with pelvic node dissection is performed on too many patients who have too much disease to hope that the operation will encompass all of their disease. (2) The Wertheim hysterectomy and node dissection or radical hysterectomy and node dissection as it is inadvisably named in the United States, focuses too much attention on the regional nodes and not enough on the primary tumor and the immediate extensions from it.

Let me first discuss the contention that too often the surgeon tries to make the Wertheim operation accomplish more than it is designed to do. It is generally agreed

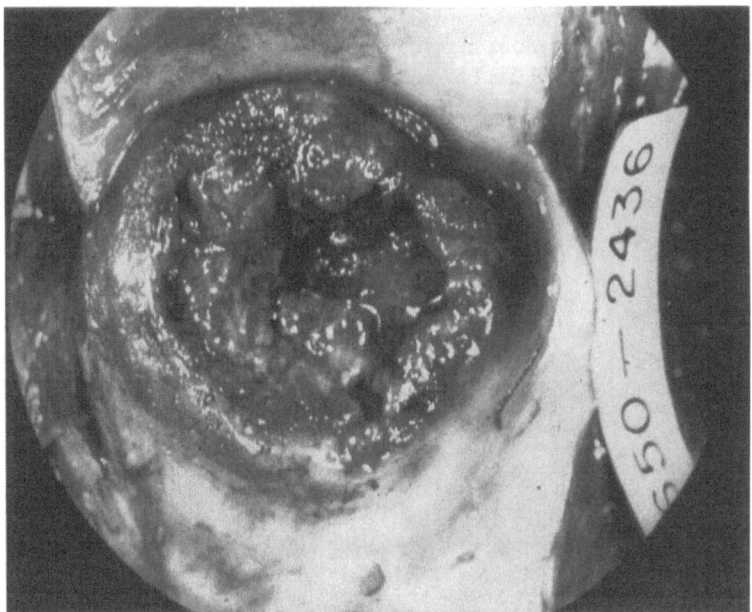

Fig. 2. Stage I. An example of the ulcerating type

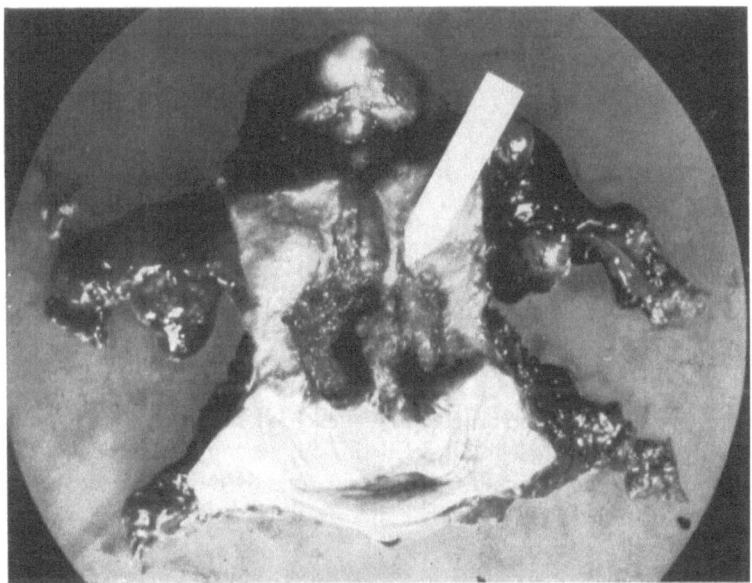

Fig. 3. Stage I. The lesion involves the endocervix

that this surgical procedure is an adequate operation for patients with the amount of disease that would place them in the categories of either Stage I or II cervical cancer. I would take issue with this statement.

In my opinion the Wertheim with pelvic node dissection gives the best results when it is restricted to patients with Stage I and IIA. The 5 year survival statistics will be less regarding when the operation is performed in patients classified as Stage IIB or III.

In evaluating my own results in patients in Stage II where the Wertheim and node dissection was done I was pleased to note a salvage rate of 67%. The 14th volume of the Annual Report notes a 53% survival for Stage II. My pleasure was short lived,

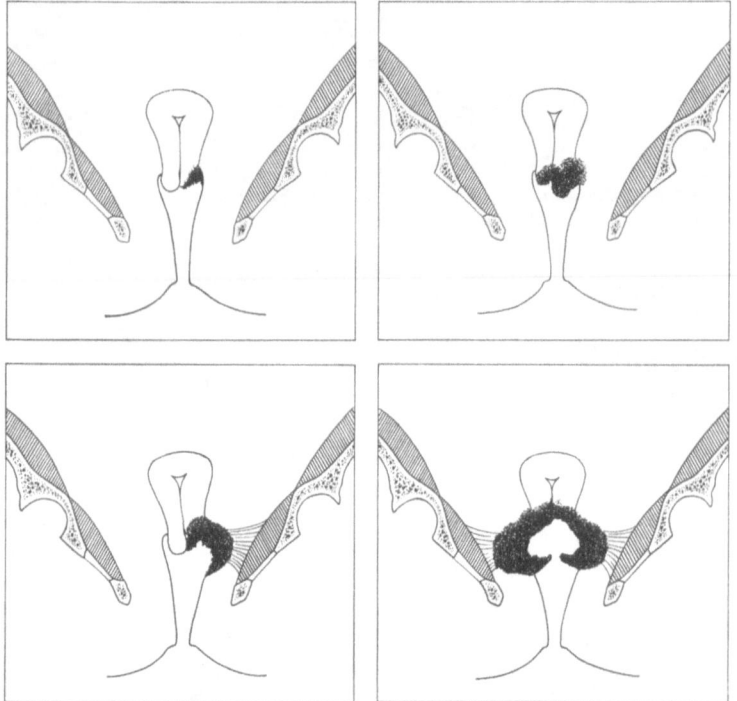

Fig. 4. Stage II. The upper portion shows the extent of the disease in the IIA classification. The lower portion shows the IIB staging

however, when closer analysis breaking down Stage II into Stage IIa and IIb that the results continued to be satisfactory in Stage IIa at 80% but fell to 43% in Stage IIb. This is what I mean about the operation being offered to patients who have too much disease to expect the Wertheim procedure will encompass all the disease and cure the patient. In my opinion if the clinical evaluation suggests more and varied disease in the IIb category that these patients should be treated by radiation, not surgery. It is not a question of technique, but rather the life history of cervical cancer and the nature of its growth pattern.

It would appear then that the Wertheim hysterectomy and pelvic node dissection has a logical but restricted place in the treatment of cervical cancer.

The next subject for consideration is the observation that some of the radical abdominal surgery is less than adequate because the emphasis in the excision is placed on the node dissection rather than on the primary tumor and its environs. In general the radical nature of the operation is judged by the extent of the node dissection. In my opinion this is in error.

No one will deny that the presence or absence of nodal metastases has a direct bearing on prognosis. We also know that patients with positive nodes can be salvaged.

In recent years there has been a tendency to shift the emphasis in therapy from the primary tumor to the regional nodes. This has been true of both surgery and radiation. The radiologist sets up arbitrary reference points at A, near the cervix and

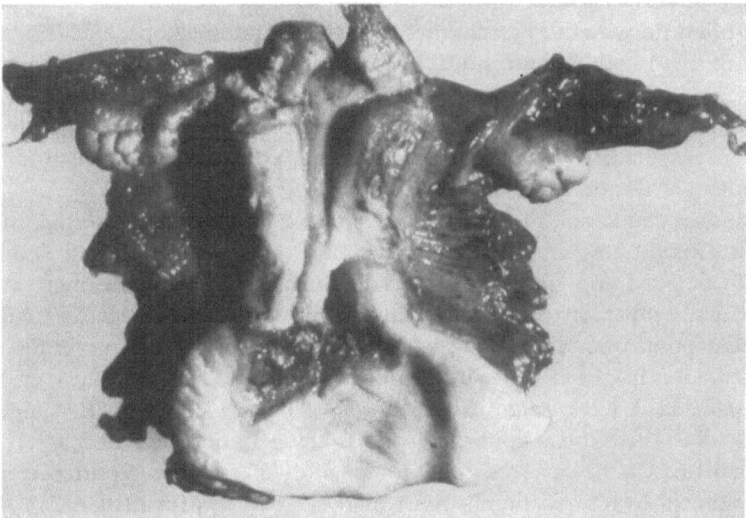

Fig. 5. Stage IIA. The cancer has left the cervix and extended to the wall of the vagina. The specimen shows the extent of the paravaginal and paracervical dissection

B, on the pelvic wall and develops elaborate dosage tables to enable him to balance the effect of the local radium and external radiation. Proper use of the tables helps him to deliver uniform without undue destruction of normal tissue or injury to bladder and rectum. Because of the doubt cast about the ability of radiation to cure metastatic nodes he concentrates on delivering radiation to the lateral areas.

The surgeon in turn, realizing that the prognosis is directly related to the extent of nodal involvement, places his emphasis on the nodal dissection and is less concerned with the vital paracervical and paravaginal area. Too much of the surgery for cancer of the cervix done in the United States today is little more than an extension of the type of hysterectomy done for benign disease with a lymphadenectomy added.

It is my contention that the success or failure of the surgical treatment of cervical cancer will depend on how well you treat the local disease and the spread to adjacent areas. The salvage figures will not improve by doing an extensive and beautiful node dissection but an inadequate excision of the tissues around the cervix.

To truly evaluate the impact of the nodal dissection on patient survival we must first have some idea of (1) how often the nodes are involved, and (2) how often the patient can be cured if they are.

How often are the nodes involved? This type of information is now becoming available as the result of the increasing experience with *Radical Surgery*. From a review of this experience it would seem to be true that the nodes are actually not involved as frequently as we have become accustomed to believe. In many instances, even when there is an extensive amount of tumor present such as we find in Stages III and IV, the patient will have no node involvement. The percentage of nodal metastases increases as the local disease becomes more advanced, but not as much as we might expect. It would be incorrect, for example, to assume that because a patient was classified as Stage III that she would certainly have positive nodes. In our experience the nodes were involved in Stage I in 14%. In Stage II the percentage of regional node metatsases was 22%. In the more advanced cases in Stages III and IV metastatic nodes were present in 36%.

How often do we cure patients with positive nodes? Approximately 50% of patients in Stage I with regional nodal involvement will survive for 5 or more years. If all patients in Stage II are included the 5 year end results will be around 35%. The chance of improving the salvage figures by the node dissection falls off sharply in the category of Stage IIb or more advanced disease. You will be fortunate indeed if 1 of 5 patients with nodal metastases survives 5 years.

It is not my contention that the regional nodes should not be dissected. In addition to the demonstrated proof that long term survival is possible when the nodes are positive in Stages I and IIa, there is an additional reason for performing a nodal excision. In all probability the patient who is reported as having negative nodes will have small deposits of carcinoma in small nodes that the pathologist never discovers. This observation has been made in relation to breast carcinoma. When the nodes were cleaned and all were examined serially a 33% higher yield of positive nodes was found. There is, therefore, a double reason for doing a node dissection.

The most recent figures from the compilation of statistics reported from the World institutes by the Radiumhemmet suggests that approximately 25% of all cervical carcinoma is in Stage I and 37% in Stage II. Only 15% of patients in Stage I have positive nodes and we salvage one half of them. Similarly 25% of Stage II cancer of the cervix will have positive nodes and the expected salvage is one in five. It would seem obvious then that the impact of the nodal dissection on the total salvage in cervical cancer is not great. The node dissections should be done, but the emphasis in therapy should be on the local tumor and the extensions from it rather than on the nodes.

Complications. If we are to shift the emphasis in treatment from the nodal and concentrate our therapy on the local area we pose problems for both the surgeon and the radiologist. Both are concerned with proper function of the bladder and intestine in the post treatment period. There is an impression that only the surgeons have complications. Recent reports in the literature suggest that serious bladder and bowel injuries have increased in number as the radiologists attempt to deliver larger doses from super voltage machines. The damage from radiation is apt to be permanent and progressive in contrast to the ureteral and vesical injuries that follow surgical intervention.

A certain number of fistulae will heal spontaneously. The remainder may pose more serious problems and require transplantation of the ureter into the bladder dome, or at times a nephrectomy. If meticulous dissections are done around the bladder the surgeon runs the risk of interrupting the blood supply to the bladder and lower ureter. In addition dissections of this magnitude impair the nerve supply to the bladder which produces the troublesome complication of bladder atony. This is more of a nuisance than a serious complication.

Fistula formation and bladder atony are technical problems inherent in any operation designed to remove all of the carcinoma. We should not fall into the trap of performing a less extensive dissection to avoid the complications and leave potential disease behind.

In past years my own fistula rate has been as high as 10%. Recently we have materially reduced the incidence of fistula formation as well as the pelvic sepsis that occasionally occurs by closing the vaginal apex and instituting catheter drainage.

The morbidity from the abdominal surgical procedures for cancer of the cervix tends to be high while the morbidity is relatively low in the neighborhood of 1%.

What about the combined use of radiation and radical abdominal surgery? The combination of radiation and surgery is being tried in a number of clinics in the United States. By combining modalities the surgeon hopes to preserve the best features of both while minimizing the complications. Such therapy may be employed in a number of different ways.

1. A preliminary trial dose of radiation is given followed by radical hysterectomy when either biopsies or vaginal smears suggest that the radiation response is unsatisfactory. If the smears and biopsies will pinpoint the radiation resistant case this will be a major contribution in the treatment of cervical cancer. Our hopes for the future rest on our ability to select the proper treatment for the individual case. As of the present time we do not have satisfactory method of making the selection although we badly need such a test.

2. In some clinics local radium therapy is routinely followed by radical abdominal surgery. In my own opinion it would appear to be more logical to carry out definitive therapy by either surgery or radiation rather than use them in combination according to a standardized plan.

3. A full course of radiation is followed by a radical abdominal hysterectomy and node dissection as part of a regular treatment program in certain clinics.

In my own experience with this approach I have found that the technical phases of the operation are not necessarily increased but there have been far too many serious injuries to the bladder. They do not appear immediately but are prone to occur after 2 or 3 weeks. It is reasonable to expect that they might for radiation has jeopardized the blood supply and surgery has added further insult. If the therapist gives less radiation or the surgeon does less of a dissection in order to minimize the damage he reduces the chance of cure. It is possible that combination therapy of this magnitude may also act as a disservice to the patient. It would seem to be unwise to have the patient go through a dangerous operation which may be unnecessary if the radiation has destroyed the tumor.

Rather than employ combination treatment in any form I would prefer to select the type of therapy which I felt best suited the needs of the patient and give it to the best of my ability.

Vaginal Surgery of Cervical Carcinoma*

E. Navratil

The use of the two basic methods, surgery and radiotherapy, either alone or in various combinations at our disposal for the treatment of epidermoid carcinoma of the cervix of the uterus enabled the introduction of a selective therapy. This form of treatment can only take into account the many individual variations of patients. One of the greatest advantages of surgery consists in the possibility of choosing one of the several types of operations providing different degrees of radicality proportionate to the stage of disease and to the individual case. Such a procedure corresponds to the aim of our treatment to make every possible effort to achieve optimal results with minimal risk to the patient. Accordingly different types of operations have been used by us when operative treatment was considered. Disregarding conizations and simple hysterectomies in the period from 1946 through 1967 without preoperative irradiation 564 Wertheim's, 989 Schauta-Amreich's operations and 56 Schauta-Amreich's

Table 1. *Epidermoid carcinoma of the cervix of the uterus. Types of radical operations. Performed 1946 to 1967 incl.*

Without preoperative irradiation			1609
Schauta-Amreich's operation	989	61.5%	
Schauta-Amreich's operation with bilateral extraperitoneal lymphadenectomy	56	3.5%	
Wertheim's operation	564	35.1%	
With preoperative irradiation			76
Schauta-Amreich's operation	23	30.3%	
Schauta-Amreich's operation with bilateral extraperitoneal lymphadenectomy	1	1.3%	
Wertheim's operation	52	68.4%	
Total			1685

operations with bilateral extraperitoneal lymphadenectomy (extended radical vaginal operation) have been performed. After preoperative irradiation 52 patients underwent the abdominal, 23 patients the radical vaginal operation and one case the extended radical vaginal operation (Table 1).

Having been asked to discuss radical vaginal surgery only, some preliminary comments may be made. The following widely accepted factors are valid reasons for the selective use of this operative procedure:

1. Patients withstand the operation much better than the Wertheim operation. Therefore the operation is rarely contraindicated on general medical grounds or advanced age. Thus the vaginal approach is used even by those operators, who generally are not in favour of it, in cases in which the Wertheim's operation is contraindicated or in cases with extreme stoutness or an associated prolapse.

---

* From the Department of Obstetrics and Gynecology, University of Graz, Graz, Austria.

2. A very low postoperative mortality and a very low incidence of postoperative complications can be claimed as one of the great advantages of the radical vaginal operation. Uretero-vaginal fistulae especially are extremely rare.

3. Follow-up examination of the patients show that late complications of the urinary tract are relatively rare.

The main argument advanced against the use of the radical vaginal operation is that it does not allow a lymphnode dissection. However, experience has proved that the end results by the Schauta operation achieved are satisfactory. In discussing the value of this procedure SHAW for instance stated, that "it is one of the puzzling features of gynecological surgery that such good figures are obtained when pelvic lymphatic glands are left undisturbed". These good results can be explained by the different incidence of lymphnode involvement in the various histological and clinical stages and by the statement again advanced by LANGDON PARSONS, CESARE and FRIEDELL that "the problem of successful management rests largely on the adequacy with which the local spread of the disease is treated. The emphasis should not be primarily on the node dissection but on the adequate excision of the paravaginal and paracervical tissue". If the vaginal operation would not satisfy this last postulate, the reported end results could not be understood. On the other hand there seems to be till now no agreement regarding the necessity of the surgical removal of the lymph-field and in regard to the therapeutic value of lymphadenectomy. Like the other advocates of the radical vaginal operation MCCLURE BROWNE believes that if the nodes are involved there is no point in the dissection and if they are not involved there is no need for it. Furthermore neither GRAHAM nor RAUSCHER and SPURNY found good evidence that the surgical removal of the lymphnodes significantly increases the 5-year survival rates. These statement would logically speak in favour of the vaginal operation. However, we do not agree to these arguments uncondi-tionally. Our attitude towards the lymphnode problem is based on the assumption that lymphadenectomy is of great importance in cases, in which in the light of our informations the incidence of lymphnode metastases can be expected to be high. That applies especially to cases of progressed Stage I and to the cases of Stage II. The same is valid for cases of all stages of disease regardless of the histologic grade of stromal invasion, if on a biopsy or on the extirpated uterus a carcinomatous lymph- or bloodvessel invasion can be demonstrated. Therefore the vaginal approach was used selectively.

The efficiency of the vaginal operation has already been substantiated by numerous reports. However, in general, they do not seem to have attracted much attention. Within the brief period still at my disposal it is therefore my intention to present our immediate postoperative results and survival rates, achieved by the Schauta-Amreich operation in cases without preoperative irradiation. Postoperative X-ray treatment was applied to the majority of cases of clinical stages, whereas in preclinical cases this treatment was omitted.

The distribution of stages and ages respectively of the 989 patients is presented in Table 2. According to our indications for the Schauta-Amreich operation the majority of cases belonged to Stage I. However, more than one third have been cases of early Stage II and some of Stage III (vagina). 10% of the patients have been older than 60 years.

In the discussion of the complications it seems justified to subdivide the whole period in the years 1947 through 1951 and 1952 through 1967, as the first 5 years represent the postwar time with various well-known difficulties. Besides that the method of the isolation of the ureter was changed in 1949. Thus for assessing actual results reference must be made to the 756 operations performed in the last 15 years.

Regarding the injuries to bladder, ureter and rectum it must be pointed out that no distinction is made between avoidable and unavoidable ones according to the spread of the carcinoma. Thus their total incidence is presented in Table 3. The majority of these lesions occurred in the first 5 years. As our experience increased their incidence was reduced considerably. The isolation of the ureter is generally considered as the crucial point of the operation. Accordingly it may be emphasized that one ureter was lacerated in only five cases (0.5%) during the course of its isolation. Among the first 233 operations a damage to one ureter occured twice (0.9%) and among the last 756 operations three times (0.4%). The bladder was injured in 16 cases (1.6%) and the rectum in one case (0.1%). In the light of these results it can be stated that the incidence of injuries to ureter, bladder and rectum is very low, providing that the vaginal approach is correctly indicated and that a satisfactory operative technique is followed. However, it can not be expected that avoidable injuries can ever be eliminated completely.

Table 2. *Schauta-Amreich operation. No preoperative irradiation. Epidermoid carcinoma 1947 to 1967 incl. Ages of 989 patients*

Age	Stage							
	I		II		III		Total	
	No. of cases	%	No. of cases	%	No. of cases	%	No. of cases	%
21—30	41	4.1	6	0.6	—	—	47	4.8
31—40	203	20.5	61	6.2	3	0.3	267	27.0
41—50	206	20.8	120	12.1	6	0.6	332	33.6
51—60	111	11.2	123	12.4	6	0.6	240	24.3
61—70	45	4.6	56	5.7	1	0.1	102	10.3
71—80	1	0.1	—	—	—	—	1	0.1
	607	61.4	366	37.0	16	1.6	989	100.0

For the evaluation of all radical hysterectomies the development of secondary fistulae, especially of the urinary tract, is of great importance. The incidence in our cases is presented in Table 4. The majority of uretero-vaginal fistulae was observed in the first 5 years. Whereas among 233 operations performed during this period seven unilateral uretero-vaginal fistulae (3.0%) developed, among the following 756 operations only one fistula (0.1%) was observed. This improvement is in our opinion due to the modified method in the isolation of the ureters described by us in the year 1949. As the incidence of other fistulas is also extremely low it can be postulated that the problem of fistulae can be practically disregarded.

Using a 30 day follow-up suggested by BRUNSCHWIG to estimate postoperative mortality, our mortality for the first 5 years was relatively high (3.4%), but for the following period only 0.8%. Thus as of today it can be assumed to be approximately 1%.

In conclusion it can be stated that the immediate results are satisfactory. However, it must be emphasized particularly that they can be evaluated correctly only in

Table 3. *Schauta–Amreich operation. No preoperative irradiation. Epidermoid carcinoma. Incidence of injuries. 1947 to 1967 incl.*

Period	No. of cases	Bladder		Ureter		Rectum		Bladder and Rectum		Total	
		No. of cases	%	No. of cases	%	No. of cases	%	No. of cases	%	No. of cases	%
1947—1951	233	7	3.0	2	0.9	—	—	—	—	9	3.9
1952—1967	756	9	1.2	3	0.4	1	0.1	1	0.1	14	1.8
1947—1967	989	16	1.6	5	0.5	1	0.1	1	0.1	23	2.3

Table 4. *Schauta–Amreich operation. No preoperative irradiation. Epidermoid carcinoma. Incidence of postoperative fistulae. 1947 to 1967 incl.*

Period	No. of cases	Bladder		Ureter		Rectum		Bladder and Rectum		Intestines		Total	
		No. of cases	%	No. of cases	%	No. of cases	%	No. of cases	%	No. of cases	%	No. of cases	%
1947—1951	233	1	0.4	7	3.0	1	0.4	—	—	—	—	9	3.9
1952—1967	756	2	0.3	1	0.1	2	0.3	—	—	2	0.3	7	0.9
1947—1967	989	3	0.3	8	0.8	3	0.3	—	—	2	0.2	16	1.6

relation to the end results achieved. The 5-year cure rate has been generally accepted for estimating the therapeutic results although this does not mean freedom from recurrence 5 years after initial treatment. Accordingly in the Annual Report the results of various institutions after periods of 7 and 10 years are published too. Thus our survival rates will be presented not only after 5 years, but also after 10 and even after 15 years. In doing so there remains to be mentioned that no distinction is made between death from carcinoma or from other disease because not every case had a postmortem examination.

The 5-year survival rates for 823 patients operated upon in the years 1947 through 1962 are summarized in Table 5. Of these cases 611 or 74.2% survived 5 years. The survival rate in 502 cases Stage I disease was 86.3%, in 306 cases Stage II 55.9% and in 15 cases Stage III (vagina) 46.7%. One case of Stage III formerly missed is living after 5 years. The survival rates for the last 10 years are presented in Table 6. They demonstrate the results achieved by our present indication for the Schauta-Amreich operation.

Table 5. *Schauta-Amreich operation. No preoperative irradiation. Epidermoid carcinoma. 5-year survival 1947 to 1962 incl.*

Stage	No. of cases	5-year survival		
		No. of cases	%	Lost sight of
I	502	433	86.3	4
II	306	171	55.9	—
III	15	7	(46.7)	—
I—III	823	611	74.2	4

For the evaluation of the 10-year cure rates 568 cases operated upon during the period 1947 through 1957 are at our disposal (Table 7). The 10-year cure rate was for these cases 63.0%. Of 323 cases of Stage I 77.1%, of 231 cases of Stage II 44.6% and of 14 cases of Stage III (vagina) 42.9% are living after 10 years.

The 15-year cure rates refer to 294 patients who had been operated upon in the years 1947 through 1952 (Table 8). Of these cases 142 or 48.3% have reached the 15-year survival date. The survival rate in 132 cases Stage I disease was 66.7%, in 151 cases Stage II 33.8% and in 11 cases Stage III 27.3%. It must be assumed that these results will be improved in the future because they are now based on operations performed in their majority in the post-war time.

Summarizing it can be expected that the reported results and the survival rates should be accepted as a proof of the efficiency of the radical vaginal operation in a selective treatment for epidermoid cervical carcinoma. There is no question, that in surgical treatment of cervical cancer the Schauta-operation will maintain its ground because there will always be cases, which are operated better by the vaginal than by the abdominal procedure and because more and more early cases will be detected, in which the dissection of the lymphnode bearing areas is unnecessary. In closing, I hope that this presentation will stimulate interest in this operative procedure and will lead to its further use.

Table 6. *Schauta–Amreich operation. No preoperative irradiation. Epidermoid carcinoma. 5 year survival. 1947 to 1952 incl. and 1953 to 1962 incl.*

Period	Stage											
	I			II			III			I–III		
	No. of cases	%	Lost sight of	No. of cases	%	Lost sight of	No. of cases	%	Lost sight of	No. of cases	%	Lost sight of
1947–1952	132/105	79.5	1	151/74	49.0	1	11/4	(36.4)	—	294/183	62.2	1
1953–1962	370/328	88.6	3	155/97	62.6	—	4/3	(75.0)	—	529/428	80.9	3

Table 8. *Schauta–Amreich operation. No preoperatioe irradiation. Epidermoid carcinoma. 5-, 10- and 15-year survival. 1947 to 1952 incl.*

Stage	No. of cases	Living at 5 years		Living at 10 years			Living at 15 years		
		No. of cases	%	No. of cases	%	Lost sight of	No. of cases	%	Lost sight of
I	132	105	79.5	95	72.0	2	88	66.7	4
II	151	74	49.0	60	39.7	—	51	33.8	2
III	11	4	(36.4)	4	(36.4)	—	3	(27.3)	1
I–III	294	183	62.2	159	54.1	2	142	48.3	7

Table 7. *Schauta-Amreich operation. No preoperative irradiation. Epidermoid carcinoma. 5- and 10-year survival 1947 to 1957 incl.*

Stage	No. of cases	Living at 5 years			Living at 10 years		
		No. of cases	%	Lost sight of	No. of cases	%	Lost sight of
I	323	275	85.1	2	249	77.1	8
II	231	124	53.7	—	103	44.6	2
III	14	6	(42.9)	—	6	(42.9)	—
I—III	568	405	71.3	2	358	63.0	10

References

GRAHAM, J. B., L. S. J. SOTTO, and F. P. PALOUCEK: Carcinoma of the cervix. Philadelphia: W. B. Saunders Co. 1962.

MAYER, H. G. K.: Geburtsh. u. Frauenheilk. **28**, 338 (1968).

McCLURE BROWNE, J. C.: Discussion. J. Obstet. Gynaec. Brit. Emp. **67**, 724 (1960).

NAVRATIL, E.: The Schauta-Amreich operation. In: MEIGS, J. V., and S. H. STURGIS, Progress in gynecology, Vol. IV. New York, London: Grune and Stratton 1963.

— Amer. J. Obstet. Gynec. **86**, 141 (1963).

— Radical vaginal hysterectomy (Schauta-Amreich operation). In: Clin. Obstet. Gynec. Vol. 8, No. 3. New York: Hoeber Med. Division. Harper and Row Publ. 1965.

PARSONS LANGDON, and G. H. FRIEDELL: The evaluation of pelvic lymphadenectomy in the treatment of cervical cancer. In: MEIGS, J. V., and S. H. STURGIS, Progress in Gynecology, Vol. IV. New York, London: Grune and Stratton 1963.

—, F. CESARE, and G. H. FRIEDELL: Surg. Gynec. Obstet. **109**, 279 (1959).

RAUSCHER, H., u. J. SPURNY: Geburtsh. u. Frauenheilk. **19**, 651 (1959).

Evaluation of Different Methods of Treatment of Cervical Carcinoma*

O. KÄSER and A. CASTAÑO Y ALMENDRAL

Cure of cancer of the cervix depends first on the nature and extent of the tumor, second to a lesser degree on the skill and experience of the therapist, and third to some extent on the modalities of treatment [21].

This could explain why the results of different methods of treatment — radiotherapy, surgery and various combinations — do not differ materially. The question then arises as to whether the different therapeutic regimes cure the same tumors and fail to do so with the others, or if their therapeutic spectrum is different thereby enabling a selective therapy to produce better results. A definitive answer cannot be given at the present time. However, experience has shown that a few persistent or recurrent carcinomas after radiotherapy can be cured by surgery and vice-versa [5, 28]. The number of these cases, however, is too small to alter the apparent 5 year recovery rate significantly. The number of cures would most likely be increased if the diagnosis of a persistent or recurrent carcinoma could be made earlier than it is possible by the now available methods.

It is well known that at the present time in most institutions about one third to one half of all cases are beyond cure at the beginning of primary therapy [27]. This

---

* Herrn Dr. H. J. WESPI, Chefarzt der Frauenklinik Aarau (CH) zum 60. Geburtstag in Freundschaft gewidmet.

situation can only be changed by earlier detection of cancer with a broad scale screening program [29, 37].

Another question which cannot be answered satisfactorily is the difference in terms of cure rates between what we consider an optimal and an inadequate surgical or radiotherapeutic treatment of cancer of the cervix. It is true that the Annual Reports [27] show improving apparent recovery rates which are probably due in part to better treatment. But it is also well known that cases have been cured after insufficient treatment, and that failures occur after seemingly adequate therapy.

Table 1 shows the 5 year apparent recovery rates of the four most important therapeutic regimes:

1. Surgery with minimal selection and so called "tailored procedures".

2. Surgery, mostly abdominal, different degrees of selection with or without pre- and/or postoperative radiotherapy.

Table 1. *5-years apparent cure rate*
(14th annual report and other sources)

	Stage I %	Stage IV %	Stage I—IV %
Surgery[a] (minimal selection)	79	20	57.4
Surgery[b] (mostly abdominal ± heavy selection)	73—84	0—5	44—64
Surgery[c] (vaginal and abdominal ± heavy selection)	72—82	0—9	54—63
Radiotherapy[d] (minimal selection)	69—86	5—12	42—59

[a] Memorial Hospital and James Ewing Hospital New York.
[b] Frankfurt, Graz, Ljubljana, St. Louis.
[c] Amsterdam, Hannover, Jena, Wuppertal.
[d] Copenhagen, Manchester, München, Stockholm.

3. Surgery, mostly vaginal or partly vaginal partly abdominal, with different degrees of selection with or without irradiation and

4. radiotherapy exclusively or with only occasional surgery.

The results shown are those of a few institutions with large numbers of cases chosen arbitrarily in the 14th Annual Report [27] or the literature [4, 19, 48]. The 5 year results for League of Nations Stage I, Stage IV and all stages combined for these four therapeutic regimes do not differ significantly. This is true also for two additional methods; the first systematic preoperative radiation [16, 17, 45], and the second systematic postradiological lymphadenectomy in advanced cases. This second method has never gained wide acceptance and has now mostly been abandoned because of a prohibitive morbidity [38].

There are of course a few "high fliers" in the literature with better results [27] but smaller numbers of patients. This fact does not prove a superiority of treatment, as it is well known, and has repeatedly been pointed out by KOTTMEIER, that results depend on many other factors [27].

The recovery rates by BRUNSCHWIG and his collaborators [47] with different surgical procedures according to stage of disease and condition of patients and minimal selection are impressive especially in Stage IV cases; but they are not superior to those with other therapeutic regimes [11, 27]. Also few other institutions have the facilities to repeat Brunschwig's surgical experiment.

We therefore come to the conclusion that presently available data and especially the lack of controlled studies do not prove the superiority of anyone of the above mentioned methods. Also according to some authors [13, 42] there is no statistically significant difference between the abdominal operation with and without lymphadenectomy.

If the data about recovery rates are inconclusive, there is, however, little doubt that for many and perhaps most cases of carcinoma of the cervix radiotherapy is the best or often the only possible form of treatment because of the size of the tumor and/or the condition of the patient. The two advantages of radiotherapy are a lower mortality — generally below 0.5% — and morbidity especially early morbidity [2, 6, 8, 10—12, 23, 24, 26, 35, 36, 40, 44]. The number of fistulas in Stages I and II is very small [26, 47].

An additional reason to favor radiotherapy has recently been given by BADIB and collaborators [3]. These authors found in autopsy cases of cancer of the cervix that modern radiotherapy had cured cancer of the cervix spreading beyond this organ more often than surgery. After radiotherapy significantly more women showed only distant metastasis and no residual cancer in the pelvis. After both methods — modern surgery and modern radiotherapy — the women survived much longer than they would have formerly. Again the number of cases is too small and the groups are not comparable statistically to prove a point.

Both methods of treatment have a significant morbidity which is higher however after surgery (and most probably higher after abdominal than after vaginal operations) than after radiotherapy. Surgical mortality has been cut down to less than 1% in many institutions [15, 24, 29, 30, 44].

In Frankfurt three patients were lost in 667 radical abdominal operations giving a primary or hospital mortality of 0.45%. The morbidity of our abdominal operations is high if asymptomatic bacteriuria is included. The rate of severe complications is not excessive however and the number of fistulas which has been lowered as in many institutions [2, 15, 24] is acceptable.

In our hospital 78% of all patients showed one or more complications (Table 2) the most frequent being bacteriuria. The number of ureteric fistulas was 21 or 3%, in the last 150 cases there were 3 or 2%. Six patients had rectal or bladder fistulas. We feel that the measures listed in Table 3 are important in order to prevent ureteric fistulas.

What then are the advantages and indications for surgery? Two important advantages are the possibility of preserving the ovaries and a functional vagina in younger women. Preservation of these structures probably does not constitute a risk for the patient and preserving these organs is becoming more important as an increasing number of young women with early lesions are being treated. For these cases (carcinoma in situ and early invasive cancer) surgery is probably the best form of treatment because its radicality can be adapted to the individual patient. After surgery these patients can be followed by cytology which is more difficult or impossible after radiotherapy.

For many authors diagnostic conization or hysterectomy in certain cases in an adequate treatment for carcinoma in situ localized to the cervix [1, 29, 37, 49]. Hysterectomy may even be adequate for early invasive cancer. The question then arises for which size of the tumor and for which additional qualities of early carcinomas — infiltration of blood or lymph vessels, histologic type, inflammation etc. — full cancer therapy — radiologic or surgical — is mandatory. This question cannot

Table 2. *Complications (% of total) in 667 Wertheim operations for cancer of the cervix (1950 to April 1968)*

Mortality	(3)	.45
Intestinal obstruction		1.6
Thrombo-embolism		4.5
Pneumonitis		2.0
Urinary tract infection		45.5[a]
Pyelonephritis		7.3
Febrile course (48 h <)		29.0
Lesions of ureter	(8)	1.2[b]
Fistulas ureter	(21)	3.0
Fistulas bladder/rectum	(6)	.9
Wound infection		
abdominal		3.5
vaginal		3.0
Wound disrupture	(2)	.3
No complications		22.0

[a] 80% with urine culture.
[b] 2 intentional sections.

Table 3. *Prevention of urinary tract damage*

1. Pre- and postoperative urography.
2. Preservation of mesureter.
3. Limited dissection of ureterovesical angle.
4. Preservation of umbilical artery.
5. Extraperitoneal suction drainage.
6. Double layer peritonealization.
7. Closed system bladder drainage.
8. No routine irradiation.

be answered satisfactorily, but it is reasonable to assume that with a tumor of less than 0.5 to 1 cm the advantages in terms of 5-year cure rates of a conservative approach; i.e. smaller mortality and of course morbidity, may outweigh its disadvantages; i.e. the possibility of lymphatic spread. It has been shown in many institutions including Frankfurt that with microcarcinomas of the cervix positive regional lymph nodes are found only very exceptionally, i.e. in less than 1 to 2% [22, 50]. Even with tumors of up to 1 cm in diameter positive nodes seem still to be rare [49, 50].

An important concern of many authors at present is the search for a "minimal effective and safe treatment" [29, 37] of the early stages of cancer of the cervix. The dangers of overtreatment of these cases are considerable at least in many European countries.

The other indications for surgery are listed in Table 4. The indications 1 to 5 are widely accepted. Radioresistent and recurrent carcinomas after radiotherapy are only exceptionally cured by a second course of ionizing agents, and the results of chemotherapy are equivocal and palliative at best [25, 41]. Therefore surgery is often the only hope of cure.

The indications 6 to 10 are not generally accepted. Probably the 5-year recovery rates of surgery and radiotherapy in these cases are more or less identical. It is possible, however, that by individualizing therapy and selecting patients for one or the other form of treatment results might be improved. But this depends on a close cooperation of the radiotherapist and the gynecologic surgeon.

The success of operative treatment of cancer of the cervix depends largely on the experience and skill of the surgeon. These qualities cannot be gained by operating the

Table 4. *Indications and possible indications for surgery in operable cases of invasive cancer of the cervix*

1. Early lesion, Stage Ia.
2. Radioresistant or recurrent tumors
3. Ca cervix and fibromyomas or ovarian tumor.
4. Ca cervix and p. i. d.
5. Ca cervix, unfavourable local conditions for radiotherapy.
6. Stage Ib to IIa cases.
7. Stage IV cases (exceptional).
8. Ca cervix and pregnancy.
9. Adenocarcinoma.
10. Ca cervix and positive nodes (lymphangiography).

exceptional radioresistant cases only. This is therefore an additional reason why surgery of primary cases should be continued.

In summarizing I would say that radiotherapy is the best form of treatment for the majority of cases examined in most institutions at the present time. On the other hand, surgery still holds an important place in treating cancer of the cervix because of its advantages, especially in younger women and in early lesions. The results of the two methods in operable cases are comparable and the complication rate of surgery is not prohibitive.

References

1. ADELMAN, H. C., and S. I. HAJDU: Amer. J. Obstet. Gynec. **98**, 173 (1967).
2. ANTOINE, T.: Med. Coll. Virg. Quart. **3**, 56 (1967).
3. BADIB, A. O.: Cancer (Philad.) **21**, 434 (1968).
4. BARBER, H. R. K.: Results of the surgical treatment of cancer of the cervix at the Memorial-James Ewing Hospital, New York. In: MARCUS, S. L., and C. C. MARCUS, Advances in obstetrics and gynecology, Vol. 1, p. 622. Baltimore: The Williams and Wilkins Company 1967.
5. —, and A. BRUNSCHWIG: Results of the surgical treatment of recurrent cancer of the cervix. In: G. C. LEWIS, New concepts in gynecological oncology. Philadelphia: F. A. Davis Company 1966.

6. BICKENBACH, W.: Med. Coll. Virg. Quart. **3**, 35 (1967).
7. BRUNSCHWIG, A.: The operations for cancer of the cervix. In: MARCUS, S. L., and C. C. MARCUS, Advances in obstetrics and gynecology, Vol. 1, p. 608. Baltimore: The Williams and Wilkins Company 1967.
8. COLPITTS, R. V.: Urologic complications encountered in the treatment of patients with squamous carcinoma of the cervix. In: Carcinoma of the uterine cervix, endometrium and ovary, p. 175. Chicago: Year Book Publ. 1962.
9. CUCCIA, C. A.: Amer. J. Roentgenol. **99**, 3711 (1967).
10. DEDDISCH, M. R.: Med. Coll. Virg. Quart. **3**, 54 (1967).
11. FLETCHER, G. H.: Radiotherapy of cancer of the cervix uteri. In: Carcinoma of the uterine cervix, endometrium and ovary, p. 69. Chicago: Year Book Publ. 1962.
12. FRIEDMAN, E. A., and H. C. TAYLOR JR.: Amer. J. Obstet. Gynec. **93**, 758 (1965).
13. FROEWIS, J.: Wien. klin. Wschr. **74**, 357 (1962).
14. GRAHAM, I.: Surg. Gynec. Obstet. **126**, 799 (1968).
15. GREEN, T. H.: Obstet. and Gynec. **28**, 1 (1966).
16. GREISS, F. C., JR.: J. Amer. med. Ass. **193**, 1105 (1965).
17. GREISS, F. C.: Combined radiation and surgical treatment for carcinoma of the uterine cervix. In: G. C. LEWIS, New concepts in gynecological oncology, p. 133. Philadelphia: F. A. Davis Company 1966.
18. —, and D. D. BLAKE: Clin. Obstet. Gynec. **10**, 567 (1967).
19. GORYS, H. P.: Zbl. Gynäk. **82**, 1561 (1960).
20. GUTTMANN, R.: J. Amer. med. Ass. **193**, 1104 (1965).
21. HAHN, G. A.: Amer. J. Obstet. Gynec. **96**, 631 (1967).
22. HILLEMANNS, H. G., u. T. KRÖPELIN: Arch. Gynäk. **204**, 42 (1967).
23. HOLZAEPFEL, I. H., and T. C. POMEROY: Amer. J. Obstet. Gynec. **97**, 625 (1967).
24. KÄSER, O.: Med. Coll. Virg. Quart. **3**, 42 (1967).
25. KARNOFSKY, D. A.: Chemotherapy of recurrent cervical cancer. In: G. C. LEWIS, New concepts in gynecological oncology, p. 171. Philadelphia: F. A. Davis Company 1966.
26. KOTTMEIER, H. L.: Complications of radiotherapy of carcinoma of the cervix. In: MARCUS, S. L., and C. C. MARCUS, Advances in obstetrics and gynecology, p. 633. Baltimore: The Williams and Wilkins Company 1967.
27.— Annual report on the results of treatment in carcinoma of the uterus and vagina. 14th Vol. Stockholm 1967.
28. — Evaluation of treatment of recurrences after surgery and radiotherapy of carcinoma of the cervix. In: G. C. LEWIS, New concepts in gynecological oncology, p. 161. Philadelphia: F. A. Davis Company 1966.
29. LATOUR, I. P. A.: Amer. J. Obstet. Gynec. **97**, 631 (1967).
30. O'LEARY, I. A., and R. E. SYMMONDS: Obstet. and Gynec. **28**, 745 (1967).
31. LOUROS, N. A.: Med. Coll. Virg. Quart. **3**, 40 (1967).
32. LUCCI, I. A.: Carcinoma of the cervix and pregnancy. In: Carcinoma of the uterine cervix, endometrium and ovary, p. 217. Chicago: Year Book Publ. 1962.
33. NOLAN, J. F.: Megavoltage radiation therapy in recurrent cancer of the uterine cervix. In: G. C. LEWIS, New concepts on gynecological oncology, p. 157. Philadelphia: F. A. Davis Company 1966.
35. PARKER, R. T.: Amer. J. Obstet. Gynec. **99**, 933 (1967).
36. ROGGE, U.: Zbl. Gynäk. **90**, 487 (1968).
37. ROMAN, T. N., and I. P. A. LATOUR: Amer. J. Obstet. Gynec. **97**, 739 (1967).
38. RUTLEDGE, F.: Experience with pelvic lymphadenectomy. In: Carcinoma of the uterine cervix, endometrium and ovary, p. 175. Chicago: Year Book Publ. 1962.
39. — J. Amer. med. Ass. **193**, 1102 (1965).
40. — The role of surgical resection in the management of cervical carcinoma. In: Carcinoma of the uterine cervix, endometrium and ovary, p. 149. Chicago: Year Book Publ. 1962.
41. SMITH, I. P., and F. RUTLEDGE: Amer. J. Obstet. Gynec. **97**, 800 (1967).
42. SPURNY, J.: Krebsarzt **13**, 401 (1958).
43. SYMMONDS, R. E.: Carcinoma of the cervix and pregnancy. In: G. C. LEWIS, New concepts in gynecological oncology, p. 181. Philadelphia: F. A. Davis Company 1966.
44. — Amer. J. Obstet. Gynec. **94**, 633 (1966).

45. Stallworthy, I. A.: Med. Coll. Virg. Quart. **3**, 45 (1967).
46. Truelsen, F.: Cancer of the cervix. London: Lewis 1949.
47. Weise, W., u. G. Reichel: Zbl. Gynäk. **83**, 1561 (1960).
48. Anselmino, K. I.: Geburtsh. u. Frauenheilk. **21**, 120 (1961).
49. Ober, K. G., u. H. Meinrenken: Gynäkologische Operationen. In: Guleke, N., u. R. Zenker, Hrsg., Allg. und spez. Chirurg. Operationslehre. 2. Aufl., Bd. IX. Berlin-Göttingen-Heidelberg-New York: Springer 1964.
50. Reiffenstuhl, G.: Das Lymphknotenproblem beim Carcinoma colli uteri etc. München-Berlin-Wien: Urban und Schwarzenberg 1967.

Diagnosis of Recurrent Carcinoma of the Cervix

Joseph H. Pratt

Nearly half of the patients with carcinoma of the cervix will eventually die of persistent or recurrent disease. If patients who do not respond to initial therapy could be identified early and positively, many of them could be cured or the course of their disease so modified as to offer significant palliation. However, for the purpose of this discussion, we must distinguish between persistent and recurrent cervical cancer. Persistent cancer is that which never disappears, and all cases should be diagnosed during the first 3 months after treatment. Recurrent tumors are those that initially heal after radiotherapy and subsequently recur locally or elsewhere. When the primary treatment involves surgical extirpation of the lesion and the margins of the wound seem to be free of tumor, any reappearance — other than immediate local reappearance — is considered a recurrence.

Our problem is to diagnose recurrences as early as possible. Since additional treatment not only carries a considerable risk but may be mutilating, the diagnosis must be as nearly unequivocal as we can establish it. This, of course, means pathologic identification of viable tumor cells. However, most carcinomas of the cervix are treated primarily with radiotherapy, and surgical meddling with vigorously irradiated tissue may lead to necrosis, complications, or the breakdown of tissue barriers. Therefore, indiscriminate or "routine" biopsies should be avoided. Only when the radiologist, clinician, or surgeon believes a lesion is not responding satisfactorily should the patient be subjected to additional biopsies.

The majority of recurrences and deaths from cervical cancer take place in the first 3 years, and this is the critical time for care and diagnosis of recurrent tumor. But even after 5 years, 3% to 5% or more of the patients will die of recurrences. The first step in a program to diagnose recurrent cancer is in the routine care of all patients after primary treatment. Gary et al. (1964), on the basis of their studies, advise examinations monthly during the first 3 months, every 2 months from 3 to 27 months, and biannually thereafter. Breen goes even further and sees his patients every 2 weeks for 3 months and every month for 2 years. At the Mayo Clinic, where our patients come from a wide geographic area, we have advised routine examination every 3 months for 1 year, twice a year for 5 years, and once 1 year thereafter. Suit et al. (1967) rather pessimistically expressed the opinion that radiation doses necessary to kill all tumor cells would have to be in excess of the amounts used clinically; thus, since there is no natural mortality of tumor cells, recurrences would be found in almost all cases, if the tumor sites were examined long enough. In a recently reported case, recurrence did appear after 30 years (Howkins and Andrews, 1955).

Our base line for the evaluation of a patient is her general health and the local pelvic findings at the conclusion of her initial course of therapy. From this point on she should improve; if she does not, then more extensive investigations rather than routine examinations are indicated. Unexplained loss of weight is significant, as is a general deterioration of strength, vitality, or physical well-being. Since the administration of radiation therapy is subject to variation and since tissue response to irradiation varies considerably, each patient must be judged on the basis of the course of her own illness, including physical findings and laboratory data.

The cervix and upper part of the vagina receive the maximal doses of radiation and are therefore less likely to be sites of *recurrent* cancer than are other parts of the vagina or the lateral pelvic tissues. Furthermore, if the upper part of the vaginal tract is free and pliable, if there is no ulceration, and if there is no induration, then there is no *local* or *central* recurrence. Any area of ulceration, of course, should be biopsied. Vaginal smears are not as satisfactory after radiation as one could wish but are helpful, and they are very good after primary surgical treatment. If a smear is positive *and the cervix and vaginal vault seem normal,* then Schiller's iodine test may help one pick a spot to biopsy. A test involving the use of a hematoporphyrin derivative may point out a precise spot to biopsy (LIPSON et al., 1964), if the necessary materials are available and if one has had sufficient experience with it. Solitary suburethral metastasis is uncommon from a cervical lesion, yet PAUNIER et al. (1967) reported 17 cases in a series of 965 in which the patients were known to have died of recurrent cervical malignancy. Biopsy and diagnosis of such lesions present no problem.

There is always some change in the pelvis after irradiation or operation. An experienced radiologist or surgeon can, hopefully, distinguish the nodular, wooden-hard, fixed tissues of recurrent cancer from the smoother lesions of radiation fibrosis. Yet mistakes can be made, either in observing the malignant tissue too long or in assuming that everything palpable is malignant. KAPLAN et al. (1965) have reported several such cases. We recently had a case which illustrates the problem. The patient, a 44 year old women with a Stage III lesion, had been treated with an adequate course of radium and X-rays. 4 months later — primarily because of a nonfunctioning left kidney but also because of a large ulcerating hemorrhagic fixed pelvic mass, anemia, and a high erythrocyte sedimentation rate — definitive operation was thought to be contraindicated. Because of brisk hemorrhage 1 month later, she was operated on, and bilateral ligation of the internal iliac arteries was done. The patient was sent home for terminal care, but she subsequently came to the Mayo Clinic. Reexploration was thought advisable, and it turned out that, after resection of the left ureter and its reimplantation into the bladder, a Wertheim type hysterectomy and node dissection were possible. Most of the pelvic fixation proved to be the result of radiation changes, necrosis, and ulceration, only an occasional clump of tumor cells being found near the ureter. One positive node was found. This patient lived comfortably and well for more than 2 years. While such cases are unusual, far too often a patient with a questionably recurrent cancer is observed until the lesion is so large and so characteristic that it has become truly unresectable and the patient is beyond hope of surgical extirpation of the cancer.

If, during a routine examination, the physician finds a palpable change in the pelvis, either a distinct nodule, a noticeable increase in fibrosis or fixation, or a lateral mass, he must obtain biopsy specimens of the responsible tissue. Sometimes this may be accomplished by means of needle biopsy through the vaginal vault, rarely trans-rectally. Frequently, it is necessary to make a small incision in the vault to reach the suspicious region. This should be done in an operating theater, as bleeding may be excessive. Also, a pathologist should be available to give a diagnosis based on examination of a frozen section. More often than not, the first specimen or two is inflammatory, but a deeper one may show malignant cells.

Another patient, a 32 year old women, had had a simple vaginal hysterectomy for what was apparently a Stage I lesion. On examination here 1 year later, a 4 cm mass was found behind the vault. The ovaries could not be identified per se. Needle biopsy through the vault confirmed recurrence of cancer. Thus, a lesion was discovered at a time when it was resectable, and a Wertheim hysterectomy was carried out. The patient has survived 10 years.

Lateral pelvic masses are most often confused with lymphocysts. The latter are rounded, hemispherical, smooth, generally nontender, and discrete; but they do *not* feel cystic on palpation. They are present early, by the third month postoperatively, they do not change in size, and they contain clear fluid. They can be explored extra-peritoneally and unroofed for biopsy. Lymphocysts should not cause ureteral obstruction; therefore, if obstruction is present, the retroperitoneal tissues should be explored further.

If the uterus remains, as after radiation therapy, and there is any change in vaginal discharge, or if the uterus seems to become larger on subsequent bimanual examinations, then dilatation and curettage of the endocervical region, as well as the fundus, is indicated to rule out spread of the malignant disease into the body of the uterus. A diagnostic Wertheim hysterectomy may be the procedure of choice if the post-treatment vagina and cervix are completely stenotic.

The patient with pelvic metastasis may develop signs or symptoms suggesting a deeper or higher recurrence. Unilateral edema frequently is the first hint of recurrence along the pelvic wall, involving the iliac or obturator region and extending behind the iliac artery and vein onto the muscles and fascia. These regions are high enough in the pelvis that pelvic examination of even a thin patient may reveal very little. Persistent sciatica, with some progression of pain, not particularly related to activities or position but present at night as well as in the daytime, is a poor prognostic symptom. In fact, after treatment for cancer of the cervix, any persistent, newly developing, localized, and not easily explained ache should alert the physician to the necessity of obtaining roentgenograms of the bones in the region of pain or even a bone scan of the pelvis and spine. Hydronephrosis and hydro-ureter also suggest recurrence of tumor. Ureteral obstruction low in the pelvis may be due to radiation fibrosis, but high ureteral obstruction, at the pelvic brim, is due almost always to recurrent cancer. The triad of edema, sciatica, and hydronephrosis must be considered as due to malignant disease, not fibrosis.

Persistent urinary tract symptoms or repeated urinary tract infections require excretory urograms and cystoscopic studies. The symptoms may result from radiation cystitis, but active cancer occasionally is found. If bullous edema is seen, the probability is great that cancer is invading the bladder wall.

Proctoscopic examinations are helpful. They permit one to observe changes in the bowel and, particularly if ulceration is present in the rectovaginal septum, to carefully obtain biopsy specimens to exclude malignant ulceration.

We do not use lymphangiograms, as they have not proven as accurate as we would like in picking out metastatically involved nodes. Ultrasonic waves may eventually prove helpful but are not diagnostic. Venography as reported by DALALI et al. (1954) is more diagnostic, especially when one is trying to distinguish between edema due to lymphatic obstruction and that due to venous obstruction. It can be attributed to venous obstruction only in the absence of adequate collaterals.

If there is a suggestion of recurrence or if the patient's symptoms are suspicious, laparotomy may be necessary to prove or disprove the diagnosis. When possible, of course, such a diagnostic procedure should be continued as definitive treatment. Unfortunately, at times even laparotomy does not answer the question conclusively, and then one can only treat the patient conservatively and optimistically. If there still is a suggestion of a central recurrence though not confirmed by biopsy and the tissues could be extirpated surgically, then the surgeon will have to decide whether to go ahead with a Wertheim or exenterative operation or to persist in further observation.

The diagnostic laparotomy is, hopefully, to exclude cancer or, if it is present, to determine its extent. The first tissues to be checked, therefore, should be the liver, the peritoneal surfaces of the upper part of the abdomen, and the omentum. Metastasis in these regions precludes definitive or radical pelvic operation. The aortic nodes should then be palpated; and, if enlarged nodes are present, one or more should be removed for diagnosis. Only then should the surgeon take the time and energy to look for recurrent cancer in the pelvic region. Retroperitoneal exploration of the iliac and obturator regions is not difficult, nor is it difficult to explore the ureters at the pelvic brim and to obtain biopsy specimens from near the ureters or even from behind the great vessels. However, when sciatica is the presenting symptom, it is extremely hard to dissect along the obturator nerve, into the iliopsoas muscle, or close enough to the sacral plexus to really exclude a deeply metastasizing cancer. When recurrent cancer has been identified, yet is unresectable, silver clips can be used to outline the extent of the recurrence.

Cervical cancer does tend to recur locally and to remain in the pelvis; therefore, we may get a second chance at it. But distant metastasis occured in 341 of 2,220 patients treated at one hospital, according to CARLSON et al. (1967). They reported that single organs were involved in 110 instances and multiple sites in 231. Affected lymph nodes, if palpable, were generally inguinal or supraclavicular; and, although these were accessible for biopsy and excision, most often multiple sites were involved. The lungs were the second commonest distant site, and one third of the pulmonary metastases were solitary. Our feeling has been that if a chest film reveals a lung nodule, we first compare it with previous films. Then we try to exclude a primary bronchogenic lesion, and finally, before excising the nodule, we wait 2 to 3 months and recheck the patient. If no evidence of additional metastases has developed, the nodule is excised (DECKER et al., 1962).

Bony metastases pose a problem in that they may give severe symptoms without providing roentgenographic evidence of their location; therefore, no confirmatory biopsy is possible. When symptoms are severe, local radiation may be tried without a definitive diagnosis.

References

BREEN, J. L.: Personal communication to the author.
CARLSON, V., L. DELCLOS, and G. H. FLETCHER: Radiology 88, 961—966 (1967).

Dalali, S. J., A. A. Plentl, and A. L. Bachman: Surg. Gynec. Obstet. **98**, 735—742 (1954).
Decker, D. G., J. W. Warren, O. T. Clagett, and D. C. Dahlin: Amer. J. Obstet. Gynec. **84**, 192—197 (1962).
Gary, R. K., J. M. Sala, and J. S. Spratt, Jr.: Radiology **83**, 208—218 (1964).
Howkins, J., and J. D. Andrews: J. Obstet. Gynaec. Brit. Emp. **62**, 870—871 (1955).
Kaplan, A. L., P. T. Hudgins, and J. A. Wall: Amer. J. Obstet. Gynec. **92**, 117—123 (1965).
Lipson, R. L., J. H. Pratt, E. J. Baldes, and M. B. Dockerty: Obstet. and Gynec. **24**, 78—84 (1964).
Paunier, J.-P., L. Delclos, and G. H. Fletcher: Radiology **88**, 555—562 (1967).
Suit, H., R. Wette, and R. Lindberg: Radiology **88**, 311—320 (1967).

Management of Recurrent Cervical Cancer

Eugene M. Bricker

In the United States in the past 20 years there has been an intensive study of the role of extended pelvic surgery in the treatment of advanced or recurrent carcinoma within the pelvis. The concept of ultraradical surgery sprang up simultaneously in several different clinics but was given impetus by the publications of Brunschwig and Appleby appearing in 1948 and 1950. Brunschwig reported his initial results of pelvic exenteration in the treatment of advanced carcinoma of the uterine cervix. Appleby reported on "proctocystectomy" in the treatment of advanced carcinoma of the rectum in males. One of Appleby's patients was a 7 year survivor of this operation, having been operated upon in 1943. My own initial excursion into this field of surgery occurred in 1940 and 1941 at the Ellis Fischel State Cancer Hospital in Columbia, Missouri, where a few patients were operated upon just before World War II. The results in these cases were not good because of poor selection of patients for the operation and because the problem of urinary diversion was not solved. These patients were never reported in the literature.

After World War II my interest in advanced pelvic cancer was resumed and a few male patients with advanced rectal cancer were operated upon successfully. It was not until after Brunschwig's report in 1948 that I became interested in advanced and recurrent cancer of the cervix and in doing pelvic exenteration on those patients who were referred to me by the gynecologists in our medical center. Since this time my colleagues and I have accumulated enough experience to enable us to crystalize our ideas regarding the indications for this type of ultraradical surgery and to allow us to give a fair estimate of the morbidity, mortality, and survival rates that may result. Our results are similar to those obtained in other medical centers, the differences in morbidity and mortality figures being chiefly an indication of the differing criteria used in the selection of patients for operation. The success of this type of surgery is dependent upon factors that pertain to both the patient's cancer and to the surgeon doing the operation. It is a biological characteristic of certain cancers of the cervix and of the rectum that they may remain localized to within the pelvis for a long period of time. Although quite large locally, with involvement of contiguous organs, there may be no regional lymphatic metastases. Such lesions theoretically are curable if operated upon radically enough. The surgeon must have judgment and skill. He must exercise judgment in the selection of patients for the ultraradical operation, in determining what is operable and what is inoperable, and he must have the necessary surgical skill to carry the rather complicated operation to a successful completion. This skill will be dependent upon adequate training and background in the various techniques of surgery involved.

An inseparable part of this clinical problem has been the development of a method of urinary diversion in the absence of a rectum. Various clinics approach this problem in different ways. The transplantation of both ureters to the remaining portion of the colon producing a so-called "wet colostomy" was the method used by BRUNSCHWIG and APPLEBY in their early cases. Bilateral skin ureterostomies were tresorted to in some patients. The use of the terminal ileum and cecum as a substitute for the urinary bladder was given a trial. During our own experience we tried several methods of substituting for the urinary bladder after pelvic exenteration but none were satisfactory until we developed the idea of transplanting the ureters to a segment of small intestine which acted merely as a conduit to convey the urine to the outside of the abdominal wall in a convenient location. We reported upon three cases of urinary diversion by this method in 1950, not realizing that essentially the same idea had been reported in the German literature by SEIFFERT in 1935, nor did we realize that MERSHEIMER and KOLARSICK were, at the time of our report, doing the same operation in laboratory dogs. The use of the ileal conduit for urinary diversion after pelvic exenteration has been so satisfactory that one of the chief objections to the operation has been removed. Indeed, the use of an ileal segment for this purpose has been widely accepted and has been used by many surgeons as the preferred method of substituting for bladder function in any age and for any reason. The acceptability of the ileal conduit is the result of the development of satisfactory external appliances that act as a receptacle for the urine when glued to the skin over the ileostomy stoma. The results of this operation have been published previously and show a most gratifying low instance of pyelonephritis (14%) and almost a complete absence of hyperchloremia and acidosis. These favorable results appear to be due to the separation of the segment from fecal contamination, the shortness of the segment which minimizes stagnation, back pressure, and ascending infection.

Selection of Patients for Operation

Since carcinoma of the cervix is the lesion most frequently requiring a decision regarding ultraradical surgery, the following comments will be limited to a consideration of this lesion. The suitability of carcinoma of the cervix for pelvic exenteration rests upon the fact that a rather high percentage of these lesions metastasize late and the patient may have advanced local carcinoma with no regional metastases. Various studies have shown that between one third and one half of the patients dying of cancer of the cervix do not have spread outside the pelvis, death having occurred from involvement of the lower urinary tract. Most of the patients that we have found to be operable have been those who have shown persistance or recurrence after irradiation therapy. Recurrence after Wertheim hysterectomy is very likely to be inoperable if the standard radical lamphadenectomy was done. The reason for inoperability in these cases is that it is impossible to get outside the previous plane of dissection and the recurrent cancer will usually be found to involve this plane. This does not mean that recurrence in the central pelvis involving the vaginal stump after hysterectomy may not be operable.

Although most of our patients have had irradiation, we feel that there is a place for ultraradical surgery as a primary method of treatment in selected patients with

Stage III and Stage IV carcinoma of the cervix. It is simply important to determine that less radical surgery will have no chance for cure and that there is indeed a chance for cure if ultraradical technique is used. We do not believe that the ultraradical technique should be used in any type of case unless the surgeon feels that there is a chance for cure by the extirpation of all tumor. In other words, we do not believe in this type of mutilating, ultraradical surgery for palliative reasons alone.

In view of the foregoing, it becomes apparent that the determination of inoperability (no chance for cure) becomes most important. All patients are very carefully searched for evidence of spread of tumor outside the pelvis. If none can be found, the patient is prepared for operation. It is most desirable that a positive histological diagnosis be made either before or at the time of operation. The adbomen and pelvis are carefully searched for evidence of metastases that would indicate no chance for cure. Special attention is paid to the paraaortic lymph nodes which are biopsied if metastatic involvement is suspected. If no spread outside the pelvis can be demonstrated, it becomes a matter of determining what is operable within the pelvis. This can be extremely difficult even for an experienced surgeon. Lateral fixation and induration can be due either to tumor or to inflammation and irradiation fibrosis. True tumor fixation to the lateral pelvis is probably incurable by any technique of removal. However, in our opinion true tumor fixation very rarely occurs, the fixation in most instances being due to irradiation fibrosis.

Determination of inoperability in the absence of remote metastases can sometimes be accomplished through a combination of subjective and physical findings. We have found most reliable to be the findings of 1. pain in the pelvis and leg on the same side showing evidence of advanced disease on physical examination; 2. edema of the leg on that side; and 3. obstruction of the corresponding ureter. These findings are so indicative of inoperability that we no longer explore patients presenting this picture.

Technique of Operation

The type of surgery being referred to here is an extended attempt at extirpation of advanced disease for which no other type of therapy can offer any hope of cure. The majority of our patients had what we refer to as a standard complete pelvic exenteration which involves the removal of all pelvic viscera and lymph nodes from the iliac blood vessels down, the levator muscles, and the perineum. This operation has been previously described and I will go into no further detail here. There are certain modifications of the operation which are done with some regularity. These modifications may be an extension of the operation by the inclusion of other abdominal viscera (cecum or small intestine) or by the inclusion of major vascular structures (iliac artery or vein). More frequently an alteration of the operation will be in the direction of preserving function. Occasionally it will be found that the entire rectum can be saved and the operation can be limited to resection of the pelvic viscera anterior to the rectum. Occasionally also, it may be found that the levator muscles and rectal stump may be saved and continuity of the intestinal tract established. In addition, in recent years, we find opportunities to preserve some degree of sexual function through vaginal reconstruction by the use of a colon segment in selected patients for whom this effort appears to be worthwhile.

The technical concept of pelvic exenteration is quite simple and is complicated by only two factors; 1. control of the lateral attachments and blood supply of the pelvic viscera during resection, and 2. the necessity for substituting for the urinary bladder.

618

Operative experience has greatly facilitated the control of lateral vascular attachments. The use of the ileal conduit has greatly simplified the matter of substituting for the urinary bladder.

Material and Results

Table 1 lists the lesions for which pelvic exenteration was done at our medical center in the 15 years between 1950 and 1965. Also listed are the operative mortality and the 5 year survival rates. Carcinoma of the cervix is by far the most frequent lesion for which this type of surgery is done.

Table 2 indicates the operative mortality broken down into 5 year time periods and demonstrating a progressive drop in mortality with improvement in the selection of patients and experience in performance of the operation.

Table 1[a]. *Exenteration of pelvic organs for advanced pelvic carcinoma, 1950 to 1965*

Indications	Number of patients	Operative mortality		5 year survival rate (based on those at risk 5 years)
A. Postirradiational carcinoma of cervix	207	16	(8%)	35%
B. Carcinoma of the:				
1) Rectum or sigmoid	43	7	(16%)	30%
2) Endometrium	12	2	(17%)	30%
3) Vagina	13	1	(8%)	
4) Bladder or urethra	6	0		
5) Ovary	8	1	(13%)	
6) Vulva or anus	5	0		
7) Small bowel	2	0		
C. Sarcoma prostate	1	1		
D. Palliative operation for cancer of cervix	2	1		
E. Irradiation necrosis	13	3	(23%)	
Total	312	32	(10%)	

[a] Tables 1—6 from KISELOW, M., H. R. BUTCHER and E. M. BRICKER, Ann. Surg. 166, 428 (1967).

Table 2. *Operative mortality rates following pelvic exenteration for carcinoma of the cervix by 5 year intervals*

Years operations performed	Number of patients	Number of operative deaths	Operative mortality rate
1950—1954	75	10	13.4%
1955—1959	78	5	6.4%
1960—1965	54	1	1.8%
Total	207	16	7.8%

Table 3. *Operative mortality rates following pelvic exenteration for all lesions*

Interval	Number of patients	Number of operative deaths	Operative mortality rate
1950 to 1960	222	26	12%
1960 to 1965	90	6	7%
Total	312	32	10%

Table 4. *Absolute survival rates of 153 patients following exenteration for carcinoma of the cervix 1950 to 1960*

Years after operation	Number of patients	Number dying	Lost to follow-up	Number alive	Absolute survival rate
2	153	66[a]	1[b]	86	56%
5	153	93[a]	7[b]	53	35%

[a] These figures include 15 operative deaths.
[b] Counted as dead.

Table 5. *Postoperative complications in 92 of 207 women after pelvic exenteration for persistent carcinoma of the cervix*[a]

Complication (postoperative)	Number of patients having each complication		Number of patients dying postoperatively	
1. Intestinal obstruction	24		6	
Treated by laparotomy		9		5
Treated without laparotomy		15		1
2. Hemorrhage	8		3	
3. Ileal stoma separation	4		1	
4. Colostomy stoma separation	2			
5. Ureteral obstruction or necrosis	3		1	
6. Fecal or urinary fistula	6			
7. Acute pyelonephritis	8		1	
8. Postoperative psychosis	4		1	
9. Wound infection, pelvic abscess, peritonitis	39			
10. Convulsions	5		1	
11. Thrombosis of iliac artery	1			
12. Thrombophlebitis	8			
13. Heart failure	2		1	
14. Cerebrovascular accident	1		1	
15. Acoustic nerve damage	2			
16. Miscellaneous (Tracheostomy, atelectasis, osteitis pubis, parotitis)	6			
Total complications	123		16	

[a] 115 patients had none, 67 had one, and 25 had more than one complication.

620

Table 3 presents the operative mortality when all lesions for which pelvic exenteration was done are included.

Table 4 presents the 2 and 5 year survival rates. Those patients surviving 2 years (56%) are considered to have had a good palliative result. Those patients not surviving 2 years include those dying of the operation and those whose lesion was probably unsuitable for the extended operation. It is this latter group that we try to minimize by the exercise of proper judgment in the selection of patients for operation. The 35% 5 year survival rate appears to more than justify the operation.

The early and late postoperative complications are included in Tables 5 and 6. The low incidence of pyelonephritis in the long term followup is particularly noteworthy.

Table 6. *Complications in 75 of 191 women who left the hospital after having had pelvic exenteration for carcinoma of the cervix*[a]

Complication (late)		Number of patients having each complication
1. Intestinal obstruction		12
Operation	10	
Tube only	2	
2. Progressive hydronephrosis requiring ileal bladder revision		3
3. Enteroperineal fistula		9
Due to recurrent carcinoma	2	
Without recurrent carcinoma	7	
4. Rectoperineal fistula		5[b]
Due to recurrent carcinoma	1	
Without recurrent carcinoma	4	
5. Pyelonephritis		12
6. Ileal stoma revision		14
7. Colostomy revision		16
8. Perineal sinus or abscess		7
9. Perineal hernia		4
10. Renal calculus		2
11. Serum hepatitis		1
12. Thrombophlebitis		1
13. Incisional hernia		1
14. Osteitis pubis		1
Total complications[c]		88

[a] 116 had no further complications referable to the operation.

[b] Rectoperineal fistulae occurred in 5 of 9 women having colo-anal anastomoses.

[c] Complications incident to recurrent cancer not included except as noted (3 and 4).

Conclusion

The treatment of advanced and recurrent carcinoma of certain pelvic viscera is now an established procedure and has been proved to provide a satisfactory 5 year salvage rate when done on properly selected patients. The lesions most suitable for this type of surgery include carcinoma of the uterus and cervix and carcinoma of the rectum. 207 patients with advanced or recurrent carcinoma of the cervix were operated upon by pelvic exenteration with an 8% mortality rate and a 35% 5 year survival rate. Satisfactory rehabilitation of these patients can be expected. The technique of the operation is varied to fit the individual case and it is possible in many instances to save rectal function, and at times, to provide a functional vaginal reconstruction.

Urinary diversion by the use of an ileal segment to act as a conduit for the urine to an external receptacle has proved to be a most advantageous method of substituting for the urinary bladder in those patients having exenteration of the pelvic organs. The low incidence of early and late complications that have followed this type of urinary diversion have given the surgeon more freedom to use ultraradical procedures when they seem indicated.

The magnitude, risk and other features of this type of surgery make it mandatory that it be done only in selected centers where there are facilities and personnel capable of developing the judgment and skill necessary to do it successfully. If this is not done, the complications, morbidity, and mortality will be prohibitive.

References

APPLEBY, L. H.: Amer. J. Surg. **79**, 57 (1950).

BRICKER, E. M.: Total exenteration of the pelvic organs. In: J. V. MEIGS, Surgical treatment of cancer of the cervix, pp. 349—374. New York: Grune & Stratton, Inc. 1954.

— The technique of ileal segment bladder substitution. In: J. V. MEIGS, Progress in gynecology, Vol. III. New York: Grune & Stratton, Inc. 1957.

— Beckeneviszeration. In: KÄSER, O., u. F. A. IKLÉ, Atlas der gynäkologischen Operationen, S. 311. Stuttgart: Thieme 1965.

— Die radikale Evisceration des Beckens für fortgeschrittene und rezidivierende Carcinome. Arch. Gynäk. **204**, 1—19 (1967).

BRUNSCHWIG, A.: Cancer (Philad.) **1**, 177—183 (1948).

— J. Amer. med. Ass. **194**, 274 (1965).

DOUGLAS, R. G., and W. J. SWEENEY: Amer. J. Obstet. Gynec. **73**, 1169 (1957).

JAFFE, B. M., E. M. BRICKER, and H. R. BUTCHER: Ann. Surg. **167**, 367 (1968).

KISELOW, M., H. R. BUTCHER, and E. M. BRICKER: Ann. Surg. **166**, 428 (1967).

MERSHEIMER, W. L., A. J. KOLARSKICK, and M. KAMMANDEL: Bull. N.Y. med. Coll. **13**, 71—77 (1950).

PARSONS, L., and G. J. FRIEDELL: Proc. nat. Cancer Conf. 5, 241 (1964).

RUTTLEDGE, F. N., and B. S. BURNS: Amer. J. Obstet. Gynec. **91**, 692 (1965).

SEIFFERT, L.: Langenbecks Arch. klin. Chir. **183**, 569—574 (1935).

SMITH, R. R., A. S. KETCHAM, and L. B. THOMAS: Cancer (Philad.) **16**, 1105 (1963).